WHOSE NEEDS COUNT?

Community Action for Health

*Written for Community Health
Initiatives Resource Unit by*

Charmian Kenner

BEDFORD SQUARE PRESS | NCVO

Published by
BEDFORD SQUARE PRESS of the
National Council for Voluntary Organisations
26 Bedford Square, London WC1B 3HU

ISBN 0 7199 1163 X

First published 1986

Typeset by Latimer Trend and Company Ltd, Plymouth
Printed and bound in England by
University Printing House, Oxford

Contents

Acknowledgements

I would like to thank the people who gave their time to be interviewed for this book, and all those who kindly offered me accommodation whilst I was visiting the projects.

I would also like to thank Monic Knight of the Community Health Initiatives Resource Unit (CHIRU) for secretarial help, Alison Watt (formerly of CHIRU) for advice and support, and Jan Smithies of CHIRU for help with the final stages of the book.

This publication was made possible by a grant from the NCVO National Westminster Bank Fund.

Charmian Kenner

Note

The research for this book was done during two main periods: some projects were visited in autumn 1984 and others in spring 1985. The report describes the projects *at the time of the visit*. For further information about these projects, or details of other community health initiatives, contact CHIRU at 26 Bedford Square, London WC1B 3HU, tel. (01) 636 4066.

Introduction

Why this book?

We begin with a brief history of the writing of this book to explain our general framework, and also give some indication of the wide range of issues and concerns that are currently being taken up by groups, projects and organisations within the community health movement.

'We' are the Community Health Initiatives Resource Unit (CHIRU), three workers who endeavour to act as a resource for a movement that is growing with great speed and tenacity. We know of the existence of thousands of community health initiatives (primarily local health groups), knowledge which both excites and overwhelms us. One obvious solution to our brief to 'promote and support community health initiatives' is to encourage other people to do so! It was for this reason that we approached the National Westminster Bank Fund for support for a book that would describe a small number of community health initiatives in sufficient detail to give people ideas about how to get their own going. We also wanted to use the book to highlight *why* community action in health is so important, and so progressive a development.

The NWBF generously agreed to finance this publication, provided we included community health initiatives that are connected with the five local development agencies that the NWBF was set up to support. These agencies are: Councils for Voluntary Service – National Association; Volunteer Bureaux; the National Association of Community Relations Councils; British Association of Settlements and Social Action Centres; and Standing Conference of Rural Community Councils.

We were quite happy to comply with this, as it helped us to devise a structure for the book. So the first stage in our selection of community health initiatives (CHIs) was to ensure that each of the five agencies had two of its initiatives described. There are, therefore, descriptions of 10 CHIs. We also wanted to cover, geographically, as much of England as possible, and as many central issues as possible.

Despite this, it remains true that the community health movement cannot be comprehensively represented in one publication. The fundamental principle of self definition of needs and interests within the movement means that each group is quite unique. This of course is one of the movement's major strengths, and allows for diversity of views, vitality and enthusiasm in the thousands of local health groups across the country.[1] People meet in their homes, community centres, tenants' organisations, GP surgeries, libraries and so on, to share and support community health needs and interests. The movement is multi-cultural and multi-racial; it covers all ages, social classes and both sexes. Some groups may campaign for improvement in various aspects of the health services. Others may share their experiences of, for example, mastectomy, and support one another in this. Others may organise keep-fit sessions in their work place, and yet others may run health courses for pensioners, women with small children, or sickle cell disease carriers or sufferers. The examples could be endless. We hope that the groups covered in this book give a flavour of the variety and extent of community health action in this country.

There is currently a move in the voluntary sector to use the term 'good practice'. It is intended to indicate that projects/agencies/organisations are setting a good example in their own field. We resist this term, as it leaves too many questions unanswered – for example, 'good' to whom, 'good' for whom, and what is 'good' and how is it measured? We leave the chapters to speak for themselves.

As we are a resource unit for the whole of the community health movement, we do not necessarily work more with well organised community development health projects than with small self-help and community health groups. We see an intrinsic value in consolidating community action in health,

2

as the sheer size of the movement must counter many health professionals' assumptions that people, particularly working class people, are not interested in health. Our strategy, therefore, has been to attempt not to encourage divisions or even a hierarchy within the movement, but rather to put initiatives in touch with each other in order to strengthen one common bond throughout the movement – an understanding of the value of a *collective* response to health. For whilst, undoubtedly, there are differences in and between community health initiatives, there are also similarities and it is important not to lose sight of these.

This collective response to health can be seen to be either an implicit or explicit criticism of the foundation of health service delivery: a foundation that asserts that people are ill because of something to do with them as *individuals*, not because of how society is organised.[2] Therefore, individuals are regarded as being ill through either germs or misfortune, not because of their class, sex, race, age, employment hazards and so on. Whilst these factors may seem to have little to do with health, there is increasing evidence to show that working class people, women, black people, older people, the unemployed and the dangerously employed suffer greater illness and higher death rates than other sectors of society who are ascribed a higher social status.[3]

Community action in health – the collective response – is therefore vital. People are now challenging the idea of individual responsibility for health, and in all sorts of different ways. This book attempts to describe some of these ways, and in so doing, reveals the many dilemmas in the whole concept of community health action in the voluntary sector. Since our framework is determined by five voluntary agencies, none of the initiatives in the book has started from within the National Health Service. Whilst it is important to remember that there are some, and that those that exist have their own set of dilemmas (worth their own book!), the bulk of initiatives are external to the NHS.

One final word before turning to the content of the book. We do not support any initiative that can be seen, of itself, to be undermining the NHS by relieving it of its statutory obligations. We do believe that CHIs, in whatever form,

3

which demonstrate a collective response to health and ill health have a lot to offer the NHS in terms of how it should improve and extend its services in the future. We hope that this book will encourage discussion and debate amongst members of CHIs and health workers alike, and that, indeed, it will encourage discussion between them.

Raising the issues

We have done our best to represent the projects in this book as accurately as possible. All of those that appear in the following chapters have sent us written information about themselves, have been visited, and have received copies of each draft for comment and change. The time and effort involved in such a procedure is not evident by reducing it to this quick summary. It is, however, a process that we believe is essential, not only because research subjects should have control over how they are documented[4], but also as a mark of respect for the innovation and courage demonstrated in those community health initiatives swimming against the tide of conventional wisdom.[5]

Issues raised

Turning now to the content of the book, the intention here is to identify one or two major themes in each chapter, as pointers to issues that are of central concern to the community health movement.

Chapter 1 deals with the issue of unemployment. Evidence of a substantial link between ill health and unemployment is being constantly strengthened by research findings.[6] Illnesses which range from feelings of social failure, through to the culmination, for some, in suicide, are emerging as a direct consequence of unemployment.[7] This, like so many of the issues covered in this book, is typically regarded by medical professionals as being beyond the medical remit. So whilst many doctors may now acknowledge that unemployment is unhealthy, it is typically not regarded as part of their work to do anything about it.[8]

The failure by health professionals to confront some of the factors affecting health and causing ill health touches on

4

fundamental debates about their role. Should health professionals actually be illness professionals, with a relatively small range of mechanical skills to apply when things go wrong in peoples' bodies, or should they be concerned to *prevent* things from going wrong? In the latter case, they would need to redraw their boundaries for practice in ways quite different from current lines.

Are health professionals the best people to be tackling issues such as unemployment? Or, for as long as health professionals – but particularly doctors – hold as much power as they do, is society dependent upon them for calling for the appropriate structural changes necessary for health? Aspects of this dilemma emerge constantly throughout the book.

Community health initiatives are not merely lay and unorthodox groups of discontented people, they are groups of people tackling real health issues in reasonable and practical ways. This chapter on unemployment is Retford Employment and Unemployment Action Centre's response to the problem, a response that transcends exhortations to 'make the most of it and learn a few new hobbies'.

In **chapter 2**, Margaret Road Neighbourhood Centre tackles the issue of mental health, and also turns to the often difficult concept of volunteering, as a means of assisting mentally distressed people through to recovery. The point is made at the beginning that the professional response to mental illness is often one of 'go and do some voluntary work – it'll keep your mind off your own problems'.

The concept of volunteering *is* difficult.[9] Many find unacceptable any suggestion of people providing a free service for which others get both pay and status. Some argue that this position is overly indulgent, and that it puts ideological correctness before the reality of many people's lives, and before the needs that arise as a consequence of living in today's unequal society. Again, like the debate about the defining of the medical remit, volunteering is a theme which weaves through the book, with different sides of the debate aired in the different community health initiatives.

The Margaret Road Neighbourhood Centre draws attention to an angle that is often neglected in the volunteering

5

debate, namely that there are roles for people to play which are useful and which therefore have positive side effects such as feeling valued by others. However, these roles would not command, by current standards, 'paid work', either because of the nature of the work or because of the frailty of the person doing the work. The approach of Margaret Road Neighbourhood Centre both to mental health and to volunteering is one that sheds fresh light on these two extremely important areas.

Chapter 3 documents two community relations councils that have established health projects to look specifically at the health and health needs of ethnic minority communities. The health needs of black and ethnic minority people are not only taken account of in these two CHIs in this book, neither are women's health needs only tackled in the following chapter. However, these needs have been highlighted as they are the CHI's *particular* focus.

The particular quandary we faced when putting the book together – of chapter titles and ordering – is reflected in the different approaches within the community health movement to the issue of segregation versus separatism. Segregation is a term used by certain elements of the movement who perceive that their health needs are being segregated from mainstream health needs. This of course means that *people* are being segregated. Black and ethnic minority people feel particularly susceptible to this as a direct consequence of racism, whereby their health needs are marginalised and deprioritised, turning the needs of ethnic minorities into the problem rather than the inadequate service delivery.[10] Other minority and/or oppressed groups feel similarly.

Conversely, within different sections of the community health movement are sectors who argue *for* a position of separatism. The distinction here is that being segregated is something that is *done* to an individual or group, whereas being separate from is a *choice* made by an oppressed group on the basis of political expediency. Ethnic minority people are fiercely critical of their segregation from mainstream health care. Some, however, argue that in order to effectively challenge that process of segregation they need to organise separately in order to retain and to generate strength.[11]

6

Both CRC projects show the connections between community health work and campaigns on health service delivery. The community health work in Tyne and Wear CRC began in 1984, and whilst the long-term aim is to bring about changes in health workers' attitudes to black and other ethnic minority people, the immediate work is concerned with building networks amongst the ethnic minority communities. This is to promote confidence and a greater health knowledge, so that communities can organise themselves to make their rightful demands on health services.

On the other hand, Camden CRC's community health work has been underway for nearly 10 years. The starting-up processes were similar to those now happening in Tyne and Wear, with the project workers immersing themselves in the communities and strengthening networks. By now, Camden CRC has gathered a considerable amount of information to back up its health policy work. The CRC can effectively demonstrate that racism within NHS institutions is affecting the health and health care of ethnic minorities. Now, however, Camden CRC looks outwards to the institutions that reproduce the racism that so clearly affects the health and health care of ethnic minorities, and consistently campaigns for changes.

Chapter 4 documents a phenomenon that is becoming increasingly familiar, that of Well Woman Clinics.[12] Taunton Well Woman Centre is one such example with an additional focus of interest: the particular health needs of women living in a *rural* area. Women across the country are arguing in their thousands that medical and health care is dominated by a male medical model that has no inherent interest in taking account of women's health needs.[13] In rural areas this lack of interest is compounded by there being fewer women doctors, by a relationship with a doctor that may be social as well as professional, and by the implications of a doctor having known a woman all her life and seeing her needs primarily in the context of her family's needs.

This particular chapter draws specific attention to the role of health professionals in community health initiatives. At one level health professionals are necessary, and sympathetic women doctors can give important help.[14] At another level, however, the contradictions in wanting help from a profession that is often opposed to the interests and health needs expressed by women, are clearly articulated. In Taunton and elsewhere, women are looking for relationships with health professionals that are not patronising, that do not trivialise disabling conditions as common female complaints, and that see women as individuals with potential beyond that of reproduction.

Moving on to **chapter 5**, a new concept is introduced – a whole neighbourhood's health, and the process whereby a community health worker assists people to define their own health needs and to then take appropriate action. Of course, one of the inherent difficulties in this approach to community health development is the possibility of raising expectations beyond available resources. Stockwell Health Project avoided many of these problems by introducing to the neighbourhood a concept that was of relevance to everyone – the planning of a new health centre. The project workers encouraged residents to decide precisely what sort of health centre they wanted, including the design of the building. They then proposed the collective result to the district health authority. In this chapter we see a different relationship with health professionals. Not, as in Taunton, where the community wants a particular service – with all of those attendant problems – but where the community want access to decision-making processes typically held by health professionals, administrators, authority officers and members alone.

This chapter describes clearly the constraints *actually* experienced when some form of democracy is campaigned for.[15] Stockwell Health Project's work has gone far beyond looking at the provision of health services, into wider community health work – drawing women in particular into health groups. This has proved to be the most productive aspect of the project's work, leading to real changes in people's lives.

In **chapter 6** we reconsider social factors and social structures that have a direct bearing on health, and yet that are too often dismissed in the health care arena. This dilemma hints at what is now a central debate amongst

8

health activists: where should the responsibility for health care – or elements of it such as health education – best be placed?[16] Would health, for example, be administered more democratically through the local authorities? Notwithstanding this debate, of equal importance, however, is the need to formally close the divide between the health and social services. So much of our health is determined by factors such as housing, the quality of local traffic routes, local education facilities, provision of home helps, and so on, that the present division between the two services makes health policies difficult to generate.

Currently, it is left to small community groups such as the Community Development Unit based at Bristol Settlement to attempt to deal with the weight of the implications of the division between, in this instance, housing provision, and the local health services. Inadequate housing in one particular tower block was causing health problems, yet there is no structure for the two arms of health and social service provision to hold hands. The account of the campaign indicates very clearly both the extent of the health problems for residents and the extent of unwieldiness and sometimes obstruction by the housing authorities. Some might argue that joint consultative committees[17], that now have three representatives from the voluntary sector, exist to address the problem. Whilst some may have made a start, the *size* of the problem alone requires both substantially more finance (not necessarily new, but reallocated), and a restructuring to close the divide between the health and social services. Successful as projects like this one in Bristol may be, the voluntary sector clearly cannot be expected to solve the volume and variety of health problems associated with social structures, single-handed.

Chapter 7 focuses on an issue dear to the hearts of most health educators – the problems associated with trying to change eating habits. The workers in Crumbles Community Café astutely make the point that change has to come from *within* people themselves. Attempts to impose new values through leaflets, posters and scare tactics simply do not work. In order to counter the weight of socialisation – much of which is generated by the vested interests of the food industry[18] – people need to become familiar with new foods first, grow to like them, and *then* think of ways to change their diets.

In **chapter 8** we move on to a sector of the community health movement that tends to attract a great deal of support from health professionals – self-help health groups. Self-help tends to be regarded by professionals as an appropriate form of health activity for people, whereby they help themselves to health and do so without constituting a threat to professional practice. Indeed in many instances, self-help is regarded as a supplement to statutory care – and sometimes as a substitute. As indicated earlier, this is not necessarily the case. Whilst there certainly are thousands of self-help groups that meet to share experiences of a common illness or disability[19], there are also self-help groups that meet because their illness or disability is not adequately provided for within the NHS. In addition to providing mutual support, such groups will often campaign for improved services.

The approach to self-help taken by the workers in the Self-Help Health Project for Northamptonshire has been one of stimulating and co-ordinating – on a county-wide basis – a network of self-help groups. Obviously all sorts of self-help health groups fall under this umbrella. What comes over as particularly unique within this project is that the workers are actually in paid employment in existing voluntary organisations: one in a council for voluntary service and one in a rural county council. Between them, in their capacity as workers in these organisations, they generated this separate project which has proven to be an extremely dynamic, self-generating and interesting model.

In the **final chapter** we turn to another issue that can in a sense be seen to be the apple of this government's eye. Like self-help, the concept of community care can be interpreted as an expectation that the voluntary sector will pick up the tab for statutory obligations – and cheaply. What in fact has been shown is that good and appropriate support for people released from long-term institutions into the community is actually expensive, certainly more expensive than the traditional institutional care.[20]

The Manchester Alliance for Community Care (MACC)

feels strongly both that community care is a 'good thing', and also that to be good it must be adequately resourced. As the concept of community care might seem to fall more appropriately into the lap of social services, we must go back to the debate about the false divide between health and social services. We also need to take account of the health consequences for *carers*, working in an unsupported and under-resourced way.[21]

The approach that MACC has taken has been one of acting as a co-ordinated pressure group for many community care schemes in the area. This again draws attention to the need for community health initiatives to have access to decision-making processes.

As the concept of community care takes a stronger hold on welfare provision, the necessity for rethinking the boundary between health and social services will become increasingly evident. Many of the people discharged into the community have chronic health problems, and their health will be affected by the quality of service provision they receive. MACC has made substantial in-roads in getting to grips with this problem – using the concepts of collectivity and pressure – and demonstrating once again that whilst some of the most innovative responses are in the voluntary sector, the voluntary sector cannot succeed on a shoe-string.

To conclude

Perhaps the most striking theme to emerge is how the boundaries around health and sickness are constantly being assessed and redrawn. This process is evident in every chapter. It signifies a major strength of the community health movement, and it gives some indication of what the movement has to offer to health professionals.

There is a tendency within the health service to insist on evaluation of community health initiatives so that they may 'prove' themselves. Whilst few would disagree with evaluation in principle, as a concept it requires explanation.[22] Firstly, the methods of research employed in medicine are based on beliefs in scientific objectivism, and value-free measurement. A growing body of literature is challenging the concept of neutrality in research, whatever its nature.

Within community health initiatives, people are arguing that all research reflects subjective judgements, but usually those of the researcher. Why not allow validity to the subjective assessments of the *researched* as well? Much of the material in this book falls into this category: people speaking for themselves about their perceptions and experiences of how community health action has helped them.

Secondly, whether it is considered useful and valid or not to attempt to measure health objectively, the methods necessary for such a process are incompatible with the activities in community health action. The methods are intrusive, disruptive, and offer little back to the research subjects. Health professionals have a great deal to learn from the community health movement, if only they will allow the community a voice.

Readers of this book more familiar with the traditional health services than with the community health movement may feel alarmed at the implications of taking the movement seriously. By seriously I mean CHIs receiving adequate, sustained funding, and the health services opening up to a system of accountability to its users. Peoples' expressed *health* needs and interests are quite clearly different to those as perceived by health professionals, and peoples' needs when they are sick are also perceived differently by health professionals. If *health* is to be taken seriously, and it is difficult to find a logic in treating rather than preventing, then resources are required.

It seems to me that changes *are* on the way. The thousands of CHIs cannot fail to have an impact. We can see changes here and there, and these represent the seeds of future growth. Rather than feel alarmed, there is a great deal to be excited about. People are starting to take health into their own hands, to exert greater control and to be more informed patients when ill. Health professionals who experience so much frustration in their practice because of the weight of social factors determining health and sickness might consider celebrating the fact that thousands of people are eager to tackle such factors. Health professionals can add their weight, and can then enjoy encounters with health service users, encounters that will be more informed, more constructive and more manageable.

Alison Watt
Formerly Development Officer,
Community Health Initiatives Resource Unit

Notes

1 Somerville, G. (ed). *Community Development in Health: Addressing the Confusions*; Report of a conference organised by the King's Fund in collaboration with the London Community Health Resource and the Community Health Initiatives Resource Unit on 13 June 1984, Kings Fund Centre, 1985 (in press).

2 Working Party of the Council of the Royal College of General Practitioners. *Health and Prevention in Primary Care. Report from General Practice 18*, RCGP, 1981.

3 Working Party on Health Inequality. *Inequalities in Health*, DHSS, 1980.

Doyal, L., Pennell, I. *The Political Economy of Health*, Pluto, 1979.

Mitchell, J. *What Is To Be Done About Illness and Health?* Penguin, 1984.

4 Roberts, H. (ed.) *Doing Feminist Research*, Routledge & Kegan Paul, 1981.

5 Rosenthal, H. 'Neighbourhood health projects – some new approaches to health and community work in parts of the United Kingdom, *Community Development Journal*, Vol. 18, No. 2, 1983.

6 Giavelle, H. S. E., Hutchinson, G. & Stern, J. 'Mortality and unemployment: a critique of Brenner's time – series analysis, *Lancet*, 26 September 1981.

Fagin, L. *Unemployment and Health in Families*, case studies based on family interviews, DHSS, 1981.

Payne, R., Warr, P. E. & Hartley, J. 'Social class and psychological ill-health during unemployment', *Social Health and Illness*, 6: 1984.

7 Unemployment and Health Study Group. *Unemployment, Health and Social Policy*, Nuffield Centre for Health, 1984.

8 Council of the Royal College of General Practitioners, *op. cit.*

9 Gordon, P. (ed.) *Professionals and Volunteers: Partners or Rivals?* Kings Fund, 1982.

13

London Edinburgh Weekend Return Group. *In and Against the State*, London Edinburgh Weekend Return Group, 1979.

10 McNaught, A. *Race and Health Care in the UK*, Polytechnic of the South Bank Centre for Administration, 1984.

Wilson A. *Finding a Voice*, Virago, 1981.

11 Gilroy, P. 'Stepping out of Babylon' in *The Empire Strikes Back: race and racism in 70s Britain*, University of Birmingham, Centre for Contemporary Cultural Studies, 1982.

For a comprehensive bibliography see: Gordon, P. & Klug F. *Racism and Discrimination in Britain. A Select Bibliography 1970–83*, Runnymeade Trust, 1984.

12 The Women's Health Information Centre maintains a list of Well Woman's Clinics across the country.

13 The Women's Health Information Centre also holds a collection of general women's health groups, and an information bank documenting women's dissatisfaction with health care.

14 Kenner, C. *No Time For Women*, Pandora Press, 1985.

Barnett, M. & Roberts, H. *Doctors and their Patients: The Social Control of Women in General Practice* in C. Smart & B. Smart (eds). *Women, Sexuality and Social Control*, Routledge and Kegan Paul, 1978.

Ehrenreich, B. & English, D. *For Her Own Good*, New York, Anchor Books, 1978.

15 The London Health Democracy Campaign has done considerable work in this area and has recently produced a Charter. Details from 157 Waterloo Road, London SE1 8XF.

16 Sheffield Health Care Strategy Group. Progressive Strategies for Health 1, and 2. Sheffield, 1983 and 1984. These are reports of two conferences where such issues were debated.

17 National Council for Voluntary Organisations. Voluntary Sector Representation on Joint Consultative Committees, Community Care Project News Sheet, NCVO, 1984.

National Association of Health Authorities in England and Wales. Index of Joint Finance Schemes, NAHA, 1982.

18 The London Food Commission, PO Box 291, London N5 1DU is collecting substantial amounts of information on the issue of vested interests of food chains.

19 The College of Health, 18 Victoria Park Square, London E2 9PF, has a register of thousands of self-help groups.

14

20 Henwood, M. & Wicks, M. *The Forgotten Army: Family Care and Elderly People*, Family Policy Studies Centre, 1984.

Heginbotham, C. *Webs and Mazes*, Centre on Environment for the Handicapped, 1984.

21 Equal Opportunities Commission. *Who Cares for the Carers?* EOC, 1982.

22 Plamping, D. 'Evaluation in Practice', in G. Somerville (comp), *Community Development in Health: Addressing the Confusions, 1985*, report of a conference organised by the Kings Fund in collaboration with the London Community Health Resource and the Community Health Initiatives Resource Unit on 13 June 1984, Kings Fund Centre, 1985.

1 *Unemployment*

The Market Place Action Centre, Retford, Notts.
Bassetlaw Volunteer Bureau

Background

Long-term unemployment can devastate people's self-confidence, and seriously affect their mental and physical health. The chance to put their skills into practice, or to learn new ones, may help unemployed people to regain their confidence. However, many volunteer bureau organisers probably do not have enough staff or enough time to deal adequately with the recent influx of unemployed volunteers. Sue Leyland, as the Bassetlaw Council for Voluntary Service worker organising volunteers from the community shop in Retford, found herself in this situation.

For one year, a special project operated from the shop, called Unemployed Volunteer Link. This was run by two people who had themselves been out of work; the aim was to give volunteers consistent support and to place them with local organisations. Such placements could lead to the volunteers getting good references from the organisations involved; in one case, volunteers at a project for homeless people later got paid employment there.

Unfortunately, the funding for Unemployed Volunteer Link has not been continued. Sue, who believes that 'unemployed volunteers should have all the support they can get', is thankful that she is now able to refer people to the Market Place Action Centre, just around the corner from the community shop. 'If the Action Centre wasn't there I don't know what we'd do. People would fall by the wayside.'

The Action Centre came about as the result of a meeting convened by Bassetlaw CVS in November 1982. Representatives from the voluntary and statutory sectors discussed

NEW PROJECT TO AID AREA JOBLESS

THE Bassetlaw Council for Voluntary Services is sponsoring a new project in Retford which aims to provide many new opportunities for the unemployed, not just in Retford, but also the surrounding rural areas.

The project, based at 24A The Square, Retford, has adopted a fresh approach to voluntary work. It does not intend to simply find tasks to occupy unemployed people, but rather it will provide opportunities for, the setting up of co-operatives or small businesses, courses and skills development. Skill

ployed can benefit. These unemployed people will use the Action Centre to acquire a new skill, exploit an idea or simply remain usefully occupied until the possibility of wage earning arrives.

The Action Centre will also arrange courses for unemployed people. These may include how to apply for a job, application form filling and interview techniques etc., non vocational courses such as weight training, art, society, rock band practice sessions and vocational courses such as joinery, motorcycle mainten-

day and Friday 9 am to 5 pm; Wednesday 9 am to 2 pm, Saturday 9 am to 1 pm

'New Project to Aid Area Jobless'
Retford Workshop and Gainsborough Times, 21 October 1983

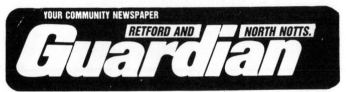

YOUR COMMUNITY NEWSPAPER

RETFORD AND   NORTH NOTTS.

Guardian

Action Centre opens new doors at Retford

by Jim Hinchliffe

IN THE LAST two months Retford Market Place Action Centre has been so successful it has already been hailed as one of the town's major assets.

About 100 people — unemployed and workers — have visited the Centre at 24a The Square and co-ordinator David Moss and his staff have listened to queries and they were pleased with it."

The list of activities the Centre could undertake was immense, said Mr Moss, but it would be enhanced if knowledgeable people volunteered to lead some of the courses. That applied particularly in arts and crafts, music, creative writing and so on.

It was hoped to introduce a women's assertive class to help those who wanted to participate more in various sections of the community but were held back by a lack of confidence.

Another course soon to be launched will deal with

technique and the completion of application forms.

Mr Newstead said many young people were nervous at interviews and did not project themselves favourably.

Mr Moss was surprised by the number of enquiries from people wishing to better their own boss. One consultative session had been organised and more were in the pipeline.

"If people show interest in any particular field we shall do our utmost to fit them up with courses," he added.

facility for group meetings and for such purposes as displaying arts and crafts and organising a book bank and workshop for community use.

Mr Newstead said the Centre was a kind of swap shop where ideas could be exchanged and people helped in many ways.

We have already seen a great deal of successful movement," he said. New doors have been opened and there are possibilities that we can help more people. Already they have

'Action Centre Opens New Doors at Retford'
Retford and North Notts Guardian, 9 November 1983
No 138

local provision for unemployed people. One suggestion was to create a new project which would offer training and, at the same time, stimulate local employment initiatives. A planning group was set up, serviced by Bassetlaw CVS and including representatives from the local authority, the

18

Trades Council, and interested voluntary and statutory organisations. A proposal for an Employment and Unemployed Action Centre was put forward to the Voluntary Projects Programme (VPP) of the Manpower Services Commission. The centre opened in September 1983, with Bassetlaw CVS acting as sponsor.

Funding

The VPP provides three full-time salaries for the Action Centre. The staff are David Moss (co-ordinator and employment initiatives officer), Jeanette Harald (education worker) and Tom Mullen (activities officer).

Objectives

The centre aims to provide 'genuine opportunities for people to develop themselves and their abilities', as explained in its information leaflet. The staff wish to help unemployed people to use their time 'constructively and enjoyably', through educational courses, training courses, and volunteer work in the community.

The Action Centre also aims to help local co-operatives and small businesses to start up or to operate more effectively.

Activities

Everyone who arrives at the centre is given a warm welcome and the chance to sit down and talk over their problems. The workers explain what the centre can offer, and suggest activities which might be particularly appropriate.

Educational courses are a key element in the programme. They range from 'Women's Assertiveness' to 'Return to Study', from 'Welfare Rights' to 'Start Your Own Business'. Many courses are run in conjunction with other bodies such as the Workers' Educational Association, (WEA), Colleges of Further Education, the Careers Service, and the Nottinghamshire Co-operatives Development Agency. A crèche is provided at the Action Centre.

The courses may be necessary as a first step towards

gaining self-confidence. One woman who came into the centre had been on tranquillisers for two years and couldn't imagine herself applying for a job. Jeanette realised that she was also too nervous of new situations to work on placement as a volunteer, so suggested instead that she should attend the assertiveness course for women.

Courses such as 'Social Awareness' and 'The Psychology of Everyday Life' have given people the chance to learn more about themselves and their mental health. Jeanette remembers the social awareness group: 'We were mainly women. We had talks on acupuncture, depression, hypnotherapy . . . a lot of information came from within the group.' The psychology course looked at topics such as: how you are affected by your family background; body language; and aggression. A parents' group, provisionally called Insight, was started. It takes a positive approach to the experience of bringing up young children: 'We want to emphasise that you can *enjoy* your child!'

The course on welfare rights provides information necessary to claim benefits, and the confidence to go out and do so. This is particularly important, because people living on benefits often feel a sense of shame – another emotionally damaging effect of unemployment. Jeanette herself experienced this when unemployed: 'You feel like a second-class citizen, intimidated. I was brought up to know my own worth, but I ended up not wanting to face another official person or fill in another form.'

David points out that the Welfare State is partly financed from National Insurance contributions, and therefore most people have paid towards their benefits in advance. However, the idea officially publicised is that many claimants are 'scroungers'. Consequently, parents who have worked all their lives sometimes will not even let their children claim benefit.

The welfare rights course emphasises that claimants are fully entitled to their benefits. The Action Centre workers encourage people to continue with their claims, despite difficulties such as long-distance travel. Jeanette notes that 'our Supplementary Benefit office is at Worksop – it's an eighteen-mile round trip. That's £2 which is two dinners'.

20

The centre offers the opportunity to do voluntary work to anybody who wishes to take it up. Some people do placements in a local organisation as part of the centre's course on 'Working in the Community'. Others get involved in projects without going on the course. Practical work done has included: building walkways through the gardens of Mount Vernon (an old people's home), helping elderly and disabled people to make their houses more secure in a 'Beat the Burglar' scheme, and doing a door-to-door Housing Needs survey. Volunteers are also encouraged to be on the rota for day-to-day office duties in the centre, such as welcoming newcomers and answering the telephone.

Many people first approach the centre for business advice. Consultants from organisations such as the Small Firms Service and the Co-op Development Agency run advice sessions at the centre. The consultants are briefed to suggest that a client takes one of the courses at the Action Centre if they think the person needs more help.

Are the objectives being achieved?

David finds that often, on arrival at the centre, 'people doubt their own abilities, they underestimate themselves'. Jeanette notes that unemployment gives a feeling that 'you're not worth counting'. For some people, even coming through the door of the centre is an achievement.

A number of people have become more confident and more enthusiastic about their lives through participating in courses or in voluntary work at the centre. On the social awareness course, for example, one woman in the group brought up a topic which concerned her – the stigma of not having children. She was encouraged by other group members to give a talk on the subject, and give support afterwards. Jeanette found that people gained enjoyment from the course as well as knowledge: 'Those sessions were great – everyone was close with one another.'

Sue Leyland of the Volunteer Bureau has seen the changes in unemployed volunteers who were initially quite withdrawn and depressed. For example, one Action Centre volunteer became 'a different person', through projects such as driving elderly people to hospital, in which he was needed and relied upon. Another volunteer, who has a stammer, helped in a door-to-door survey on housing needs. Several people on the Community course have gained the confidence to apply for other jobs and have got them. One unemployed person went on to train as a nurse after following a programme at a local hospital. Jeanette sees the centre working as 'a stepping-stone for people to come back into the community'.

Business advice sessions at the centre have been very successful. In the first year there were around eight hundred enquiries from people wanting to run their own business. Five community enterprises started with the Action Centre's support. David points out that 'setting up co-ops must be good for people – it means they have control over their own destiny'.

Lessons learned

There is a specific policy *not* to make the centre an open-door drop-in, on the grounds that people feel more constructive if they come in for a particular activity at a specified time. This approach has worked well. It also avoids the development of a clique of people who might take the centre over as a club, which could put others off using it.

However, the Action Centre has perhaps tended to reach only the more outgoing of unemployed people. At an early stage, one volunteer wanted to involve more people: he went to the pub and press-ganged a few friends! One of those people stayed on. Perhaps the centre needs to go out to make its services known, in places such as pubs and health clinics. Those who *have* come in sometimes already possess the skills on offer; almost everyone who has asked for a tutorial on interview techniques hasn't needed it.

The courses, which David and Jeanette see as a particularly important aspect of the centre's work, have not always been well attended. It may be that people lack the confidence to come. Most people have not been encouraged to see self-development as important, and they may not understand what the Action Centre could do for them.

Women seem more enthusiastic than men about coming on courses at the centre. The psychology course, for example, was attended entirely by women. Jeanette's explanation is that 'men think certain subjects are only for women. They feel out of their depth if anything's emotive.' She also points out that men don't think they should be spending time on personal discussions: their role is to earn money or to look for a job. Their self-esteem is tied up with their work, and if they remain unemployed they cannot admit to the emotional problems which result.

The welfare rights course attracted mainly women, which could be because it is often women who sort out the family's practical needs. Jeanette and David would like to encourage both sexes to come on the educational courses and learn from discussions about their lives and relationships. They are hoping that the new parents' group, Insight, will be mixed.

The Action Centre is concerned with developing new, healthier approaches to work and leisure. This task goes beyond the traditional approach to voluntary work for the unemployed, and the centre aims to help people to fulfil their own potential, by finding activities and paid jobs which suit them.

2 *Mental Health*

Margaret Road, Neighbourhood Centre,
Cullercoats
North Tyneside Volunteer Bureau

Background

Many volunteer bureaux receive volunteers sent by social
workers, GPs or psychiatrists. The people concerned may
have been through bereavement, divorce, stress at work, or
family problems. They may be feeling hurt, anxious, depressed and lacking in confidence.

The North Tyneside Volunteer Bureau can involve such
volunteers in the Margaret Road Neighbourhood Centre, a
base for self-help groups on mental health issues. Volunteers
have the chance to help other people at the centre. At the
same time, they can look at their own difficulties and try to
solve them.

Cynthia Cooke of North Tyneside Volunteer Bureau was
one of those who set up the Margaret Road Centre. She was
aware of the need to help 'difficult-to-place' volunteers, and
she was also in contact with self-help groups. When a self-
help group on schizophrenia was formed on North Tyneside, Cynthia brought in volunteers to welcome people and
act as hosts. As the group became established, the volunteers
retreated into the background. They were seen as friends,
not outsiders.

Cynthia felt that it could be useful to bring together a
range of people who all had connections with mental health
problems: volunteers who had experience of working with
the mentally ill, people who were recovering from mental
illness and would like to do voluntary work, and people
suffering from mental illness.

The Margaret Road Centre had previously been used by
Whitley Bay Social Services Department, run by a com-

munity development officer as a neighbourhood shop offering welfare rights advice and a space for meetings. The premises opened on a voluntary basis in the autumn of 1980 with a steering committee. When the centre was threatened with closure due to expenditure cuts, the volunteers took over management in 1981.

A group of volunteers, some of whom had experienced mental illness, met together to make plans for the centre. One person, George, who was manic-depressive, put forward many ideas. After a long and traumatic experience of mental hospitals, he wanted Margaret Road to be a place where people were treated sensitively. Everyone should feel welcome, and any' problems arising should be talked over calmly, without causing upsetting scenes. Cynthia describes him as 'a man with a lot of positive ideas about "care in the community"'.

It became clear that the centre would concentrate on improving people's mental health, especially via open-door listening services and self-help groups. A constitution was written, clarifying the centre's aims. Cynthia feels that 'in development work, the usual thing is to set up a structure first, then recruit volunteers. I think it's more appropriate to gather the people together and then find a structure which fits.'

Funding

The local authority provides the Neighbourhood Centre building rent-free, and gives a grant for heating and telephone bills. The centre was painted, and a carpet put in, with a grant from the Opportunities for Volunteering Scheme. The Northern Schizophrenia Fellowship, which runs groups at the centre, provides some funds, and covers some transport costs for people wanting to attend groups. Other fund-raising work is done by the centre itself, and by self-help groups which meet there, such as the group for schizophrenia sufferers and their relatives.

Objectives

Margaret Road Neighbourhood Centre aims to bring volunteers together to offer 'a caring environment to people with a range of personal and social needs'. This includes anyone feeling lonely, worried or depressed; those recovering from mental illness; and housebound and elderly people who need a friendly meeting place. The centre intends to give support and encouragement to all these people, and to improve the quality of their lives. It also hopes to foster the growth of groups with like-minded objectives.

Activities

The Neighbourhood Centre looks like somebody's front room, with comfortable armchairs, a flowered carpet and net curtains. The atmosphere is warm and welcoming, with people sitting in small groups, chatting and laughing, or just reading quietly or talking to a friend. When you want tea or coffee or a sandwich, you go into the little kitchen to make it, as if you were at home.

To encourage people to come to the centre, the 'Open

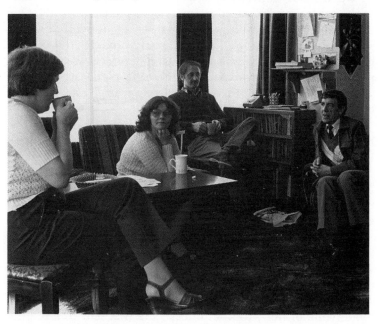

Main room, Margaret Road Neighbourhood Centre

Door' phone-in and drop-in has been publicised on the Tyneside Metro and the radio. Open Door sessions happen several times a week at the centre. One or two volunteers are always on hand to look out for new people, welcome them and offer counselling if necessary. So far these have been the volunteers who have not been mentally ill, but others are now becoming involved too. This has partly happened as a result of a Workers' Educational Association (WEA) listening/counselling course, provided at the centre at the request of a number of volunteers who wanted to train to be better listeners. Cynthia finds that for people under stress, 'listening is often 75 per cent helpful. People suffering from mental illness realise that they have to listen sometimes too.' The WEA course went well, with everyone participating openly. Trust within the group was aided by the fact that people already knew each other and were meeting in a familiar place. The group leader made sure that everyone took responsibility for listening to others during the sessions.

'Open Door' callers are told about the groups which meet at the centre, and often join one relevant to their needs. One particularly successful group was set up for agoraphobia sufferers. Agoraphobia – fear of going outside – is quite a common problem, which more usually affects women than men. A sufferer can experience horrific panic attacks: one woman collapsed in the street, feeling as if she had lost control of her body.

Some people with agoraphobia go to hospital day centres, but are not usually encouraged to meet as a group there. Cynthia felt that they needed time for themselves. She made contacts at day centres and arranged an evening meeting at Margaret Road; those who wanted to come were offered transport and collected from home. The success of that evening led to the formation of a regular self-help group.

When agoraphobia sufferers phone the Open Door service, they can have the comfort of talking to someone else who has the same problem and *has* managed to get out to the centre. One woman came to Margaret Road with her mother, who took her to work every day. She was terrified to tell anyone of her problem in case she was sent to a mental hospital. Another woman came by bus, shaking. Her need to get help at the centre was so great that she had faced up to her hatred of public transport. A man arrived by car, brought by a health visitor. Another sufferer went out to ask him in, and he couldn't believe that someone else had actually experienced the same thing.

At the self-help group, people take it in turns to talk informally, and often find that the traumas in their lives have been similar. Group members work on a programme for recovery suggested in Clare Weeks' book, *Peace from Nervous Suffering* (Angus and R, 1981). Each person is supported by a volunteer who has also read the book, and who can accompany them out into the street until they can manage to go out by themselves. One group member arrived at the centre one day saying 'I'd never have believed I could get out of bed this morning – but I did, and I walked through Whitley Bay.' By this point, people are only a step away from ordinary life. One possibility might be to come part-time to Margaret Road and go part-time to a sheltered workshop in another part of town.

A number of other groups meet at Margaret Road. One began as a single parents' group, to break down isolation. Now it has become a general women's group, in which married women and single women meet together. Group members can help each other out: for example, the married women can often babysit for the single women.

There is also a befriending group for housebound elderly people: other users of the centre often go along to help with the group's activities. Cynthia remembers a summer bus trip which was 'a riot': 'Everyone came – the Friends of the Elderly, the women's group . . . there were wheelchairs and prams . . . people helped each other out in whatever way they could.'

The Margaret Road Centre is constantly in use. Activities such as crafts, pool and table tennis, and classes in art therapy and classical guitar, are on offer. A woman living across the road from the centre makes lunch for everyone on Fridays; she used to be a professional cook. Her husband, who is a stroke patient, comes with her.

Two carers' groups are being planned to meet at the centre: one for those caring for elderly people with senile

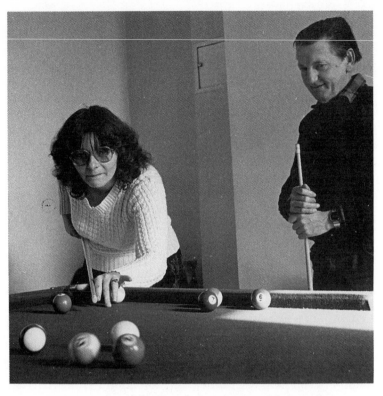

Playing pool at Margaret Road Neighbourhood Centre

dementia and another in connection with physically and mentally handicapped people. Voluntary organisations such as Action for Epilepsy and the Cancer Support Group use the centre for meetings.

The centre is always open on Sunday afternoons between 2 and 4, with tea and cakes provided. Ever since George, one of the original volunteers, emphasised that Sundays are the worst time for loneliness and depression, it has been recognised that this friendly base is of vital importance.

Are the objectives being achieved?

Many people have benefited from the opportunities for support and friendship found at the Neighbourhood Centre.

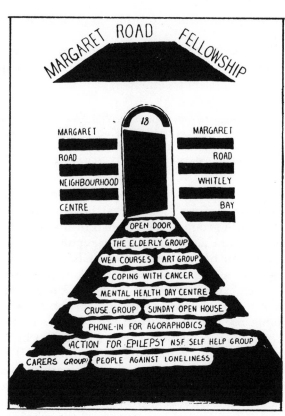

Poster designed by Caroline Gage, printed by Community Press

Dave, who suffers from agoraphobia, remembers the relief of arriving at Margaret Road for the first time:

> I didn't just feel 100 per cent better when I walked through the door. I felt 1,000 per cent better! It's like a warm understanding family here. Nobody looks at you as if you're strange. It's not like a day centre – you don't have to do occupational therapy all the time.

Change is often achieved as people get to know each other and form natural friendships. Two people may have complementary strengths and weaknesses: each can help the other to overcome a particular problem. As one parent of a schizophrenic daughter said: 'You need a one-to-one rela-

31

tionship to help someone to progress. Hospitals just don't have that.'

People who suffer from the same problem can support one another. Dave explains how the agoraphobia self-help group came off tranquillisers together:

> We're all completely off them now. You have to do it slowly, and sometimes you get terrible nightmares. When someone else in the group was going through that I could say, yes that happened to me too, but don't worry, you *will* get through it.

An unusual form of mutual help occurred at the PALS group (People Against Loneliness) held at the centre on Friday nights. A group of men from Turning Point, a hostel for recovery from alcoholism, came regularly to the meetings, as did some of the members of a CRUSE group (which helps people after bereavement). The combination of younger men, some of whom had lost their own homes through drinking problems, and older women who had a more stable background, turned out well for both groups. Some people had probably expected PALS to be a singles club, but they found something very different. There was good communication and insight into each others' needs: the men from Turning Point had learned to use Transactional Analysis during their stay at the hostel, and some were able to use this counselling technique to help the people they met at PALS. The group had some nights out dancing at a local pub. Being a large party of friends, they were not so concerned about what onlookers might think about older women and younger men dancing together.

Self-help groups have enabled members to learn more about mental illness and its treatment. Some members of the schizophrenia self-help group have become critical of psychiatrists for giving out so many drugs. They may ask their doctor 'How am I doing – can I cut down on the drugs?' or say 'I'd rather have an hour talking about my feelings.'

Bill's daughter has had schizophrenia for twelve and a half years. Bill checked in a medical book to find out about the drugs being given to her. He became concerned about the effect of Largactyl, since his daughter's face looked yellow, as if she might be getting jaundice. He initiated a long discussion on Largactyl with her doctor. Next time his daughter came home from hospital, the dose had been reduced from four tablets to three every day. Eventually it went down to nothing. After this, Bill's daughter told him that the 'voices' she used to hear were gone: perhaps they had been connected with the medication?

Bill reads many medical textbooks and recently said that he didn't want a psychiatrist to talk at the next self-help group meeting. Instead, he gave the talk himself, accompanied by pages of notes. 'I might get shot down by the doctors for reading about glands, but I believe it's right that everyone should know more about their body.' He would like to tape his talk so that other groups could use it.

Lessons learned

The success of Margaret Road depends on people meeting together on an equal basis, and helping one another by drawing on their personal experience. It can be a good feeling to find that the person sitting next to you is not a psychiatrist paid to talk to you, but a caring volunteer – someone quite like yourself, in fact. Cynthia says 'We don't have a professional approach, we just have a caring approach.' However, the centre has good relationships with social workers and health visitors. Professional back-up is available from a social worker with responsibility for mental health, but so far it has not been necessary.

The Neighbourhood Centre is meeting gaps in social service provision. As one helper, Helen, says: 'Once people are discharged from day centres there's no after-care at all – it's very sad. This is a half-way house.' Some people who come to Margaret Road live in local authority hostels. Others – several schizophrenia sufferers, for example – are living three to a room in boarding houses in Whitley Bay, with their landladies being paid by Social Services. Yet more people are referred from other institutions with paid staff, on the grounds that they are causing too much trouble. For all these people, the centre becomes the mainstay of their social life, which is left essentially unprovided for by the statutory services. Social workers who have visited the centre are impressed by its work. The centre's problem, however, is lack of money. The Northern Schizophrenia Fellowship has been providing some funds, but now this organisation itself is having problems getting its grant renewed.

It has been proved to be important that the volunteers do most of the running of the centre themselves. At an earlier stage, the Management Committee consisted mainly of people from outside. The day-to-day users of the centre gradually became more confident and ready to take on more responsibility. In preparation for a public meeting at which elections for a new management committee were to be held, the volunteers did a role-play to practise being assertive. One volunteer kept on saying, 'I think it's the people who do the work who should manage the place.' At the meeting, a committee consisting largely of volunteers was elected, by an audience composed of users of the centre. One volunteer who has trade union experience became the secretary. Volunteers now hold meetings before management committee meetings, so that any problems can be voiced at once. This helps to sort out disagreements quickly, which is vital to keeping the atmosphere healthy. Users are also encouraged to feel responsible for the centre; everyone tidies up and locks up as if it is their own place.

Not everyone at Margaret Road makes enormous or rapid progress. Sometimes a group contains too many depressed people, and despite the efforts of others to cheer them up, the atmosphere remains heavy and static. Problems arise when a person seems to have an 'investment' in being ill; they find that they can get attention that way, and if they constantly join different groups, such attention will be renewed. But the centre has more successes than failures. It shows the value of including people with mental health problems in the community, rather than separating them from others who are supposedly 'normal'. As Cynthia says, 'the line between being OK and not OK is a very narrow one', and the centre's users prefer to describe themselves as 'nervous' rather than 'mentally ill'. Everyone at Margaret Road has the potential to help others and to benefit from receiving help themselves.

3   The Health of Ethnic Minority Communities

Community Health Project, Newcastle
Tyne and Wear Community Relations Council

Background

Ethnic minority people in Britain often have to live in bad housing and work in hazardous, low-paid jobs. Many experience language difficulties and racial harassment. Women, in particular, can become isolated at home.

These conditions can cause considerable health problems. Extra health services may be needed, but these are rarely provided. Within the existing services, ethnic minority clients often encounter racist attitudes.

Tyne and Wear Community Relations Council would like to see Newcastle Health Authority do more to cater for the needs of ethnic minority groups. As Hari Shukla, senior community relations officer at Tyne and Wear CRC, says: 'We have paper after paper on the needs of ethnic minority groups. We all know the problems. But what can we do to *solve* them?' Meanwhile, the health authority runs occasional in-service training sessions on cultural differences and racism. Hospitals in Newcastle are becoming more aware that Asian people need different diets, but still tend to ask the patients' families to bring in food. Newcastle Health Authority employs one part-time liaison worker for ethnic minorities, to cover the whole area.

In order to put the case for change more strongly, the community relations council is gathering information on health problems directly from local communities. This is being done via a research and action project on community health. Two workers were appointed in the summer of 1984: Uma Mandel, to work with the Bangladeshi community, and

Lucinda Li, to work with the Chinese and Vietnamese communities.

Reports from the project workers will eventually be submitted to the health authority, and should act as a catalyst to bring about practical initiatives from the health services.

Funding

The four-year project is financed by Inner City Partnership through Newcastle Health Authority. Hari Shukla, senior community relations officer, considers that a key factor in obtaining the funding was that the proposal was submitted jointly by the CRC, Newcastle Community Health Council, and the Inner City Forum (based at Newcastle CVS).

> It's been a partnership between us all. The feeling is 'let's share' – there's a lot of expertise available. In other places, perhaps, a CRC and CVS stay apart, they speak to each other over a wall, but here we are as one.

The CRC had specialised knowledge of the communities involved, but found that the other organisations could give valuable help in formulating ideas for the health project. In particular, the CHC (of which Hari was a member for seven years) had important contacts with the health authority. Hari points out that 'If the CHC backs us up, then the health authority thinks "It's not only the CRC saying this, our own public want it too."' This broad-based support may have convinced the health authority to allocate money for a project specifically for ethnic minority communities.

Objectives

The community health project aims to identify health needs of the local Bangladeshi community and of the Chinese and Vietnamese communities. This information will be presented to the health authority, along with specific suggestions on how health services can be improved to meet the needs discovered. An equally important part of the community health workers' brief is to stimulate the development of self-help groups within the communities themselves. The members of such groups could become better informed about health, and could put forward their ideas on changes required in the NHS.

Activities

Home visits

The project workers can begin to find out what the needs of the communities are by visiting people's homes. Home visits also lead to contact with more families by word of mouth. Uma Mandel describes home visiting:

> We go and chat – we don't write lots of things down the first time. We talk about everything to do with health – food, family planning, immunisation, heating, housing. You don't have to ask much – they will bring up everything in conversation.

Many Bangladeshi people live in one particular area, Newcastle 4, and Uma concentrates her work on this district. Clinics and playgroups can provide contacts with families. Uma's task is made easier because Bangladeshi community leaders called a meeting to introduce her, explaining that she was employed to help with health matters. The Chinese community is larger and more loosely-knit. Lucinda Li started her search for families with help from the North-East Chinese Association and the Chinese school in Newcastle.

Many Bangladeshi men came to Britain twenty or thirty years ago, to work in factories, mills and restaurants. They have only recently been able to bring their families to this country. Most Chinese people have been living in Tyneside for longer, but Vietnamese families have come very recently.

Despite differences in background and history, certain similarities can be found between members of the three communities: many work in restaurants, have a low income and poor housing. As Uma says, 'When we visit we find that the health problem is not the main problem – often, it's the housing.' Children, parents and grandparents are crowded into a few rooms. They may have applied for alternative accommodation; often nothing has been done. Some families have been offered accommodation in a different area, but do not wish to move away from their community due to the fear of being lonely elsewhere.

37

Uma sees problems such as aches and pains, and coughs and colds, due to dampness, condensation and lack of heating. People's expectations of improvement in their housing are low: 'They think there's no point in asking.'

Although living conditions for Chinese families are generally better, Lucinda has come across a couple of appalling cases: families with no hot water, outside toilets and leaking roofs.

Another problem is racial harassment. Uma knows of a number of places where people have had to board up their windows because of attacks on their homes. Often families are too scared to tell the police or the housing officer of their problems.

Language difficulties are a major obstacle to use of the health services, especially for women. Uma knows of women who have to wait for someone to take them to the clinic and explain their needs. Often they only go 'in extreme necessity'. Lucinda finds that Chinese women speak little English, and Chinese men also have difficulty in communicating with doctors. There are very few Bengali-speaking doctors and even fewer Chinese health workers in the area. A Chinese health visitor was employed for a short while but has now left. Thus professionals find it hard to explain what is wrong when a client is ill, or they may not know what the client wants from them.

Women have told Lucinda that they would like doctors and nurses to be more patient with them. Several women have been told off for asking for night calls. After several hours, if no doctor arrives, they may go to the hospital – where someone else tells them off. Often they cannot describe their problem adequately in English. One Chinese woman, whose new-born baby was vomiting, rang the baby clinic, not knowing where it was or how to get there. The doctor refused to come out, and finally she rang a friend who took her to the clinic. She had a further wait in the surgery. Lucinda says, 'It was painful for the mother . . . if they could just understand a bit more.'

Uma recognises that GPs are overworked because of cutbacks, and do not have enough time for consultations. But both workers feel that doctors could· adopt a more reassuring way of talking, and could listen to people's worries more carefully. As Lucinda points out, 'Normally the ethnic minorities don't go to the doctor for little things – only if they're desperate. If they're not taken seriously, they lose faith.'

Sometimes problems arise because of differences in cultural background between the patient and the health professional. Some Bangladeshi children aged two still do not eat solids. This could be because Bangladeshi women are unfamiliar with the food they come across in this country, including canned foods, and are concerned about religious requirements such as Halal meat preparation. Advice given by a health visitor who does not understand these reasons will probably not help. The Chinese community, most of whom come from Hong Kong, are more Westernised and observe fewer restrictions on food.

Bangladeshi women usually do not wish to be examined by a male doctor, since this would be unacceptable in their own country. Uma met one tearful woman, newly arrived in England, who was pregnant and having great problems finding a woman doctor. Embarrassment can also keep women away from other facilities: keep-fit might be good for health, but, as Uma points out, 'You can't do keep-fit in a sari, and your husband might not approve if you change your way of dressing.'

Liaising with agencies on behalf of clients

Where possible, Lucinda and Uma try to help the families to solve housing problems, to claim welfare benefits, to sort out immigration difficulties, and to use the appropriate health services. Both workers spend a considerable amount of time filling in forms, writing letters and contacting officials from the relevant agencies. This work can be frustrating. For example, the Housing Department are unwilling to rehouse one Chinese family, who live in private rented accommodation, saying that they are not homeless. The defects in their housing could be put right, since it is the owner's responsibility. But the owner might not visit for a year, and the family cannot contact him.

In Lucinda's experience, the Housing Department is often not aware of the problems faced by ethnic minority people. One Vietnamese family was burgled four times within a few months, and the burglars vandalised their house, pouring tomato ketchup, flour and sauces all round the kitchen. The family gave up trying to keep the house tidy, and went to stay with relations. When Lucinda visited with the housing officer, he commented on the poor state of the house. When the Vietnamese tenants are rehoused, they will not get an extra allowance for decorating their new place if they have been blamed as 'bad tenants'. Lucinda would like officials to 'put themselves in the situation of other people – to have goodwill'.

Interpreting

There is a vast need for interpreters to help people to use health facilities. Uma is constantly called upon to act as an interpreter in clinics and hospitals. The CRC is helping a group of unemployed people to set up in business as interpreters and translators. But if people cannot afford to pay, they will continue to ask Uma and Lucinda. Another possibility is that the health authority may employ interpreters; a medically trained interpreter is being advertised for at the moment, but the health authority is having difficulty in finding applicants. Will anyone with medical training want to change their job? Uma's personal opinion is that medical training may not be necessary: 'The main need is for someone to communicate.' Adequate provision of interpreters still seems a long way off.

Group work

Parveen Akhtar of the CRC comments on the need for group work in the community health project:

> In our communities, we don't often see what I'd call 'self-help in the white context' – where groups take up an issue which concerns them. Help goes on at a more individual level, instead of through active community organisations.

In talking to families, Lucinda and Uma find that relatives

40

and neighbours sometimes help each other, but only on a limited basis. Many women are so occupied with their own families and housework that they do not have time to do things for others. Lucinda notes that some women don't want to bother other people: 'They worry that they'll resent it deep inside.' She gives the example of a Chinese woman in appalling housing, who did not tell anyone when her rent went up and she was unable to pay: 'She was afraid of losing face in the community. She just sat tight inside. People want to preserve their integrity.'

The project workers hope that groups can break down isolation and encourage women to support one another. Groups can also provide a more stimulating environment, with a range of different ideas being put forward on health topics.

Uma has started working with a group which is already in existence. Parents of children at a playgroup meet together to learn English. Everyone lives nearby, and the playgroup is an encouragement to come. For one session each week, Uma leads the group in a discussion on health issues, and invites everyone to suggest subjects of interest. A health visitor is

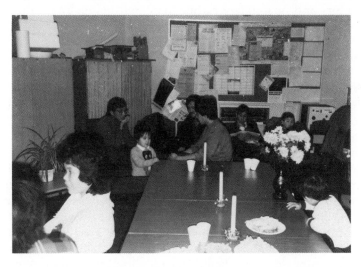

Chinese Health Group, Community Health Project,
Tyne and Wear Community Relations Council

also present. Topics have included nutrition, for which Uma used health education leaflets, translated and adapted.

Lucinda first has the task of setting up a group. She has chosen Sunday afternoons as the best time; Chinese take-away shops are closed, and children are at the Chinese school. After visiting women at home and encouraging them to come, Lucinda began the meetings. 'I myself call it the health group, but I don't say that because it would be too restrictive in their mind. I want to have a variety of subjects. I try to gently bring in some talk about diet and introduce ideas like keep-fit.' Lucinda finds that people are willing to talk about their children, and about experiences such as unsatisfactory treatment by a doctor – in which case someone else in the group may suggest a good doctor. Women can talk to her privately about subjects such as family planning or marriage problems. Hopefully, in the future these areas will be discussed in the group sessions.

Both project workers want to encourage women to look at different aspects of their lives and find out how their health is being affected. Lucinda notes that 'when we talk about health, people straight away connect to the medical side – doctors and hospitals – rather than well-being. It's difficult for us to break into that.'

Health education materials

Standard health education materials have been adapted for the project's use. Some are produced in Asian languages, but not in Chinese. Uma and Lucinda do their own translations, basing them on the original leaflets. They often find it necessary to rearrange the information to make it clearer. Both have made their own teaching charts, using pictures from leaflets. Many people are not used to reading leaflets, and are more likely to look at wall posters. Uma has begun using her own posters at her health group sessions.

Materials officially produced in Asian languages almost all concern pregnancy and child care. Lucinda and Uma identify a number of other health topics which they think would be relevant to women in their communities, including back pain, sciatica, osteomalacia, gynaecological illnesses, thrush

42

and cystitis. Other health projects in Newcastle have made their own materials on subjects like pre-menstrual tension and the menopause; these could be translated if necessary.

Are the objectives being achieved?

The project is at an early stage, but the workers have already begun to tackle all the tasks described in the initial proposal. A significant amount of information has been collected about the health problems of each community. Self-help groups have started, enabling women to meet each other and obtain health information. In the future, the groups may be able to voice their own opinions on improvements needed in the health services.

Lessons learned

The community health workers need support, since their job is very demanding. There is a support group for Lucinda and Uma, so that the workers have a place to express their feelings, doubts and problems. The Health Working Group, a part of Newcastle Inner City Forum, is represented on the support group and can supply information about similar projects already going on in the city.

Lucinda welcomes help from others: 'It is difficult for us to feel our way on our own at the beginning – they can give us clarification.' Uma feels that 'We have to have someone behind us. And we can learn from other projects – their good ideas, their mistakes.'

After only a few months in post, the project workers have come across numerous problems; how can these best be tackled? One possibility would be to concentrate on becoming welfare rights workers, taking up individual cases. However, this could lead to Uma and Lucinda being overwhelmed with casework, which is very time-consuming.

It may be better to spread information about other advice agencies, but although there are many in Newcastle, they too suffer from the language problem. Organisations such as the CRC and community associations could not cope with a sudden influx of individual enquiries either.

Group work seems a more practical method for the project

to adopt. Uma and Lucinda have started working with women, who are easier to contact at home and who are usually responsible for health issues in the family. Within ethnic community associations, which are by and large male-dominated, women usually have very little influence over issues discussed and decisions made. They tend to feel apprehensive in talking to male leaders about their personal problems and needs.

Women need the chance to talk by themselves first. After women's groups have been meeting for some time, perhaps public meetings can be arranged and men can be invited for discussion on the issues raised. Some topics, such as contraception, are particularly difficult to deal with in mixed groups, and definitely require to be approached in a women-only situation first.

Hopefully women will start to gain confidence, to become more involved in community organisations, and eventually to come forward as leaders. Uma is worried that self-help will prove hard to get off the ground, but 'we'll keep putting the points in front of them'. Lucinda thinks someone needs to take the initiative, and make some practical suggestions. For example, there could be a rota for women in the neighbourhood to look after each other's children. 'A plan may fail once, twice or three times but in the end it will succeed. It's just time that will make the difference.'

Community Health Work and NHS Policy
Camden Committee for Community Relations

Background

The National Health Service often fails to provide services needed by ethnic minority communities. For example, instead of making sure that interpreters are available at clinics, some health service officials argue that all clients should learn English. In this way, the responsibility for shortcomings in the service is shifted away from health authorities on to ethnic minority communities.

Some health service managers claim that they are open-minded in their attitude towards ethnic minority workers: 'We employ lots of black people – so what's the problem?' However, ethnic minority people are over-represented in lower-paid jobs in the NHS, and many encounter racist attitudes as they go about their daily work.

Camden CCR is campaigning consistently for changes in local health service policy, both on service provision and on employment. Chris Adamson, Community Relations Officer, points out that the NHS is a very large and significant public organisation; if it fulfils its responsibilities towards ethnic minority people, this can support the growth of anti-racist attitudes in the whole community. Community relations councils have tended to work in the first instance with local authorities, 'who are now responding in some cases'. Perhaps it is time to focus attention on other major employers.

Ethnic minority people in Camden need significant improvements in health services, as shown by the community health work which has been underway at CCCR over the last 10 years. In 1975, CCCR recognised that there were considerable health and nutritional problems amongst Bengali people in Camden. Hasmat Ara Begum was appointed as community health worker in 1976, to work primarily with Bengali women. She set up self-help groups, where women could discuss health topics and find out more about the health services available. She also contacted health workers, to raise their awareness about the needs of Bengali families.

Hasmat has become involved in health policy issues, drawing on the knowledge gained from her work in the community to point out specific policy changes which would be beneficial to Bengali people. Other CCCR workers have taken part in the campaign on health service policy. Sue Penny, appointed as deputy Community Relations Officer in

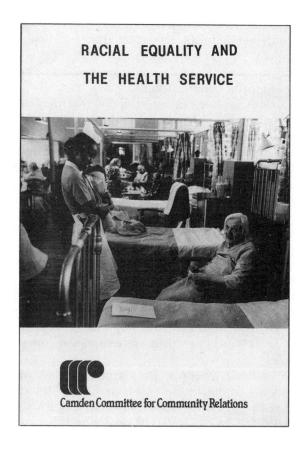

RACIAL EQUALITY AND
THE HEALTH SERVICE

Camden Committee for Community Relations

1979, spent about half her time on health policy, often working in conjunction with Hasmat. She prepared a report, *Racial Equality and the Health Service*, published by CCCR in March 1983. Chris Adamson, as CRO, is one of the people now carrying the work forward.

Funding

CCR employees have worked on health policy as part of their jobs. The first two years of Hasmat Begum's community health work were funded by War on Want and the Community Relations Commission. From May 1978 onwards, funding was taken over by Camden Council, with a smaller proportion provided by the area health authority. Hasmat is, however, based at CCCR.

Objectives

The aim of CCCR's health policy work is to campaign against racial discrimination and disadvantage in the NHS, both in its provision of health care and in its role as employer. It is hoped to stimulate the local district health authorities to combat this disadvantage.

The community health work aims to encourage Asian women in Camden to use all the facilities of the NHS, to offer them practical advice on health, and to support the development of self-help groups. A further aim is to enable CCCR to make more confident recommendations to the appropriate authorities on what could be done to deal with the problems of racial disadvantage.

Activities

Contacts between CCCR and the health service

Before the report, *Racial Equality and the Health Service*, was written, CCCR had been in touch with Camden and Islington Health Authority on the issues involved. An informal dialogue had been maintained via meetings with the chairman of the health authority, a district administrator, and sympathetic nursing officers.

47

The report was published just as new health authorities were being formed in the recent NHS reorganisation. It seemed a good moment to press for a commitment to equal opportunities for ethnic minority people.

Meetings were arranged with the district administrator of Hampstead Health Authority. During 1984, CCCR workers have given talks at training sessions for managers in this health authority, with the aim of tackling racial discrimination in the workplace. Such sessions might develop into a full training programme in the future, but this would require formal commitment at a higher level in the administration.

CCCR met with the chairman of Bloomsbury Health Authority, which then started a working party on equal opportunities in employment. Members include representatives from CCCR, the NHS and black community organisations. The health authority has decided to employ a worker on a short-term contract, to draw up a statement on the steps to be taken to promote equal opportunities. This person will work closely with CCCR, and consider points raised in the report on racial equality.

Bloomsbury Health Authority also has an equal access working party to look at service provision, with a similar range of representation. Asian, Chinese and Afro-Caribbean community organisations are amongst those involved. This group makes visits to hospitals – for example, to maternity units – to talk to staff and find out how ethnic minority people are treated.

Camden Community Health Council has an ethnic minority sub-group, which Hasmat Begum attends. Hasmat has also been a member of the Family Practitioner Committee for the past two years.

Campaigning on service provision

Staff training CCCR workers occasionally give talks to nurses, health visitors, GP trainees and medical social workers. Sometimes a small group comes to visit Hasmat at CCCR. Hasmat finds that many questions raised by NHS workers stem from ignorance. For example, nurses in one group wanted to know why some Bengali mothers breast-feed for so long. They did not realise that Bengali women are unfamiliar with foods in this country and are unsure about which solid foods can be given to babies. On another occasion, health visitors asked why some Bengali mothers did not come to clinic sessions. Hasmat described the racial harassment which Bengali women may experience if they go out of the house.

Hasmat feels that it is usually easier for the community health worker to speak at training sessions and represent the views of women who come to self-help groups. The women themselves find it difficult to attend official meetings, since they often have small children and responsibilities at home, and lack transport. Also, they might encounter strong racial prejudice from health workers. Hasmat is prepared to tackle this herself, but is unwilling to subject other women to it.

> Once three GP trainees came to a women's group. Instead of wanting to know about the problems facing the women, they started saying 'why don't you learn English?' and 'why doesn't the Bengali High Commission pay for interpreters?'

Interpreters There is an enormous need for interpreters for Camden's health services. A recent survey on maternity services in Bloomsbury Health Authority showed that many women did not go to clinics because they did not think they would be able to communicate with the staff. In practice, staff tend to ask another worker in the hospital to interpret, which may not be satisfactory. A health visitor making a home visit cannot even do this.

Hasmat used to do interpreting work, but had to stop, because the demand was overwhelming: 'I used to get phone calls day and night – I couldn't cope any more.' The work was time-consuming, because it also involved being an advocate for the patients' rights, and waiting hours at the hospital to make sure they received the care they needed. Two women from self-help groups used to work as interpreters, unpaid, but they also found the work very difficult, especially since they both had young children.

Chris Adamson thinks that CCCR cannot take on the responsibility of providing interpreters: the health service must do it. 'If you can't communicate with people, how can you start to deliver health care?'

Health information Hasmat sees the need for leaflets about clinic services to be translated into different languages, and to state when an interpreter will be present, 'otherwise women just won't go'. Health services need to be advertised more widely. Leaflets would be more likely to reach Asian women via Hasmat or via community centres.

Hasmat is happy to translate leaflets, and would like more clinics to take up this offer. She has also written her own leaflets, for example on simple dietary advice. One health visitor photocopied them for her own use. Hasmat would ideally like to work with health visitors to write leaflets, 'otherwise they might suggest food which is very healthy, but which Bengali women never eat'.

Extra services Hasmat's work has identified services which the health authorities could provide. When she was first employed, Hasmat was invited to be present at a weekly child health session in one clinic, to give advice to any Bengali women who came. Now she helps with a women's group which meets twice a week in the Family Health Clinic premises in the Middlesex Hospital. It is a comfortable room and a crèche worker is present. A health visitor sometimes comes to answer questions and films are shown on health topics. Many women also go to the Family Health Clinic itself, which operates on another day, encouraged by their familiarity with the location. This idea could usefully be extended, with women's groups meeting in other hospitals or health centres.

Hasmat would like to see Well Woman Clinics for Asian women, especially for breast checks, cervical cancer screening and gynaecological services. These would probably be best sited in the community, perhaps at health clinics. They would need special advertising, because some Asian women are not familiar with the idea of screening.

Campaigning on employment

Employment policies Chris Adamson points out that, in order to recruit ethnic minority people to the better-paid jobs, 'managers will actually have to change the way they act

50

instead of just having a paper policy'. Ethnic minority applications tend to be wrongly dismissed as 'over-qualified' or 'under-qualified'. If there is a genuine problem with qualifications, access courses could be provided to give the necessary training. This is already done in other areas such as social work. Hasmat notes that the idea of 'qualifications' should be extended to take into account all relevant abilities, such as speaking other languages.

The practice of equal opportunities in employment must be carefully monitored. As Chris says, 'Until it is clear that unless black people are appointed there will be serious problems – nothing happens.' Employing more ethnic minority people, for example as health visitors, could give clients more confidence in the NHS. Chris thinks that 'people have got to be employed who have some relationship with the people they're working with'.

The racial prejudice encountered by ethnic minority workers in the health service must be countered by making it clear that complaints will be taken seriously and dealt with. Experience in local authorities shows that as soon as ethnic minority workers feel they have the right to raise such problems, large numbers come forward.

Advertising of vacancies The CCCR report states that jobs should be advertised in the ethnic minority press. Hasmat saw an advertisement for a Bengali GP in an ethnic minority paper, with a closing date a few days later. She raised the matter via CCCR. Health authorities will obviously have to show a firmer commitment to this policy.

Are the objectives being achieved?

Over the past 10 years, Hasmat has noticed significant changes within the health services, regarding attitudes towards ethnic minority people. 'They didn't think about ethnic minorities before; they weren't aware.' Practical results are gradually being achieved.

Bloomsbury Health Authority employs three interpreters, as a direct result of pressure from Hasmat and other community workers. Hasmat's community work has also shown the need for Asian women to see a woman doctor. After a year of lobbying the Family Practitioner Committee, a Bengali woman doctor was recently appointed to a local GP practice. The ethnic minorities group of the Community Health Council is arranging a meeting with her, to discuss the community's needs and to offer her support. Meanwhile, in hospitals, 'when we ask for women to be examined by a woman doctor, they don't think it's a strange request any more'. Diets in hospitals are being improved to meet the needs of ethnic minority people, and more leaflets are being translated.

Health workers are more open towards Hasmat now. 'At first, GPs and nursing officers wanted to know my qualifications. They wondered if I was qualified to advise on diet. People wouldn't ask now.' As health visitors realised that Hasmat could help them with problems about language and culture, many became friendly. 'I know there's a balance – some people are open-minded and others not. The open-minded people make it possible to change things.' Chris Adamson, when giving talks on community relations to health service field workers, has also found a positive response. Many would like to have more black colleagues.

The report, *Racial Equality and the Health Service*, has proved a useful statement of CCCR's views, which can now be discussed more clearly with policy-makers. Chris comments that 'It's certainly started a debate.'

Lessons learned

The campaign at CCCR has shown the importance of health policy work being done in conjunction with a community health worker. Hasmat feels that 'because of working at a grass-roots level, I have more opportunities to know people's needs'. She also puts ideas into practice and finds out what the practical problems are.

Hasmat is now the only CCCR worker whose brief is to deal with health matters. She finds it a heavy responsibility, reading papers, planning for working parties and attending many evening meetings. She also finds herself reminding other workers in CCCR that health issues are important. Should another worker be appointed in this area? If another post is created, should it be for a community health worker

52

or a policy worker? Hasmat thinks that there would be advantages in having two community health workers, who also dealt with policy, because 'you can't separate the work out. Otherwise the policy-makers aren't actually hearing what people want.'

Should the NHS appoint race relations officers? Chris thinks that it is helpful to have someone with significant managerial authority: 'someone who devotes 100 per cent of their time to race relations, then the issue doesn't go away'. Hasmat is sceptical, since people who start working for the health authorities are sometimes no longer prepared to criticise NHS policy.

Should the NHS appoint community health workers? It might be better for community workers to remain outside the NHS at present, based in an organisation which can give them appropriate support. However, the NHS could fund them, in the same way as it contributes to Hasmat's salary at present.

The NHS has proved a difficult organisation to influence. A local authority, having councillors directly elected by local people, is more accountable to the public. Professionalism is often a barrier between health service workers and their clients. Chris finds that progress is very slow: 'Nothing has actually gone wrong, but it's hard to move a massive bureaucracy in which many people are unaware of the issues.'

The process of change may prove similar to that seen in local authorities. First comes a period of consultation between NHS officials, CCCR officers and local organisations. Gradually, ethnic minority community groups will become familiar with the workings of the NHS, and will keep in touch with new developments. If something happens which affects ethnic minority people, their organisations will respond immediately. Chris says:

> More and more people will gain confidence and feel they can effect change. Instead of the NHS being a part of British life that they've got to deal with, it will have to change to help them.

CCCR's responsibility is to keep the lines of communication open between the NHS and the community, until that confidence has been developed.

4 *Women's Health*

Taunton Well Woman Centre
Community Council for Somerset

Background

Women living in rural areas can find themselves in particular
need of a Well Woman Centre, where they can see a woman
doctor for a check-up or to discuss personal problems. Jenny
Mayor, who has been involved in setting up a Well Woman
Centre in Taunton, Somerset, gives several reasons for this
need.

Firstly, there tends to be a lack of women doctors locally.
For example, although most group practices in Taunton
itself now have one woman doctor, the registers are often
full. In areas outside the town, the selection of GPs is even
more restricted.

Secondly, women in smaller communities often know
their doctor socially. Whilst people want a doctor who is
sympathetic, they do not necessarily want someone who is a
friend. Women may feel too embarrassed to go for an
internal examination, for example.

Finally, when a doctor has known a woman for her whole
life, often having assisted at her birth and then delivered her
children:

> The doctor may be overly conscious of the family's needs and
> not of that woman as a woman – he sees her as 'Joe Bloggs'
> daughter-in-law' or he says 'Come on Mary, pull yourself
> together, you're a sensible girl.'

One service which can be offered at a Well Woman Centre
is cervical smear testing. Somerset has one of the highest
rates of cervical cancer in the country. Research by St
Thomas' Hospital suggests that deaths from cervical cancer
are usually due either to inadequate treatment, or to 'slow-

ness by sufferers in seeking medical help'. Women can face particular difficulties in getting smear tests in rural areas. In Somerset, many local women requested smear tests after seeing a film on cervical cancer. The Pathology Laboratory asked for such films not to be shown because they could not cope with the response.

In 1980, Somerset Area Health Authority received 'a 76-signature petition from ladies in Yeovil, relating to Well Woman Clinics'. The area medical committee recommended that 'because of the unproven value of screening for cervical and breast cancer, Well Woman Clinics should not be established'. In 1981, the area health authority again refused to open a Well Woman Centre because it saw no 'proven need'. However, in September 1981, West Somerset Community Health Council called a public meeting on the issue, which was attended by over two hundred women! After hearing speakers from Exeter Well Woman Centre, the audience worked in small groups to produce suggestions for a local centre. A steering committee was established, to set up a Well Woman Centre for Somerset.

Liz Barnes, who was assistant director of the Community Council for Somerset, had given some initial help to the campaign. She comments that:

> Well Woman Centres are one of those 'hidden needs' which are not universally accepted by funding agencies or by the medical profession. The backing of well-established local community organisations can help when a centre is being set up.

She was for a time an observer on the Community Health Council. Somerset RCC has always encouraged active members of voluntary organisations to stand for election to the CHC. Liz had thus been able to advise Jenny Mayor, who wanted to represent a post-natal support group, on how to become a CHC member. As part of her CHC work, Jenny introduced the idea of a Well Woman Centre.

Once the steering committee had been set up, the RCC magazine publicised its progress and urged readers to go to meetings. Liz says that

> We helped in small ways where we could, rather than giving formal backing. An RCC could take a more directly suppor-

tive role, particularly where they have evidence of the need for a centre.

Funding and Resources

The steering committee received administrative support from staff at West Somerset Community Health Council, who provided help with publicity, secretarial back-up, a place for meetings, services for mailing and photocopying, and information about who to approach in the health service and how to write formal letters. The district community physician was also sympathetic, and helped the committee to present the proposed budget for the Well Woman Centre to the area health authority.

The area health authority offered free use of premises, and the district community physician helped to book space in a clinic in the centre of Taunton for one afternoon a week. However, the AHA was not prepared to pay for a doctor for the centre. The Well Woman Centre supporters were left with the task of raising a considerable amount of money to pay a doctor's salary and administrative costs. With great energy, they embarked on projects ranging from coffee mornings to selling menstrual calendars at 10p each, from bazaars attended by the mayoress of Taunton to sponsored bike rides. In one year they managed to collect £1,000 – about half the annual running costs. Fund-raising has continued, since the health authority has not yet agreed to provide funding.

Objectives

The Well Woman Centre has been set up to enable women to see a woman doctor to discuss any problems which are causing them concern. The centre aims to provide a relaxed and welcoming atmosphere, and to offer information about health matters and about other relevant organisations. Decisions about the way the centre runs are taken by its users.

Activities

The Well Woman Centre sessions take place every Friday afternoon from 2pm–4pm at Tower Lane Clinic. The clinic

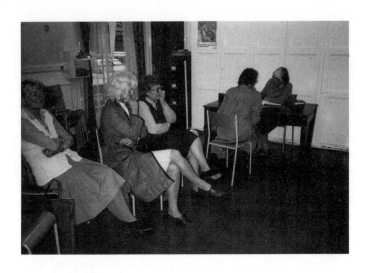

Women registering on arrival at Taunton Well Woman
Centre

door is kept wide open, so that women looking in can see the
friendly circle of chairs in the waiting area. Each person is
greeted on arrival by one of the volunteers, asked to register
at the desk and offered a cup of tea. In order to make the
centre as accessible as possible, there is no appointments
system. Women are seen in the order in which they arrive.

Numbers vary from session to session, from a few women
to as many as 13. As one helper, Cynthia, says 'I came here
one week and there was nobody, next week we had so many
we didn't know what to do with them all.' The doctor always
gives full attention to each person, and carries on until
everyone has been seen. Occasionally, if a session is very
crowded, the helpers ask whether anyone is able to come the
following week instead. If someone has far to travel home,
other clients may be asked whether she can go before them.

On purpose, no magazines have been placed in the waiting
area. Jenny says 'This has been quite a topic for discussion –
but we think that people often use them as barriers. We try
to make waiting time productive and relaxed, and give
women a chance to think about what they want to say.' The
presence of children, playing with the toys provided and

58

supervised by one of the volunteers, often leads people to make amused comments and start a conversation with one another. Volunteers chat to women as they arrive, asking whether they have come far, and how they heard about the centre; showing people the scrapbook with press cuttings on the history of the centre; and asking whether they would like to be involved in the support committee or future fund-raising activities. If women want further information about health topics, volunteers point out the leaflets available on a table at one side. If anyone wants to know about local self-help groups or advice centres, volunteers can refer to a card index on the reception desk.

Three volunteers are on the rota each week: one a committee member, another nominated by the voluntary organisation Inner Wheel, and one from a pool of people who want to help. When a new helper comes, they always work with two more experienced volunteers. The 'Hints for Helpers' leaflet lists the practical jobs that need to be done, and emphasises that the central task is 'to make the women who come to the Well Woman Centre very welcome'. Volunteers start off with jobs like making tea and doing registration, and begin talking to clients when they feel ready to do so.

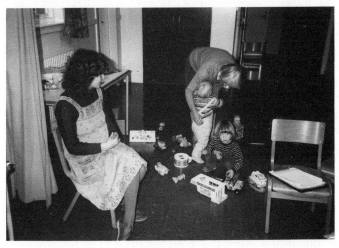

Volunteer helpers looking after children at Taunton
Well Woman Centre

Volunteers do not get special training and do not do individual counselling. At an early stage in the planning, some members of the campaign felt worried about lay women taking on a counselling role, although this method is used in other Well Woman Centres.

Most women come to the Well Woman Centre alone, but some are accompanied by a friend. Friends can go in with them to see the doctor, or wait. Sometimes a man phones up to say that he feels worried about his wife's health, and to ask if she can come. One woman was brought to the centre by her husband; once she had relaxed, volunteers suggested that he go shopping whilst she saw the doctor. Sometimes mothers want to go in with teenage daughters. If it seems important for the daughter to have privacy during the discussion, the doctor may suggest that the parent leaves.

Everything which is said between a woman and the doctor is kept confidential. The doctor does not prescribe treatment, although she can do internal examinations and tests. She has remarked that it's quite liberating not to write prescriptions, but to concentrate on talking with women instead. She can, however, with the woman's consent, telephone a GP if she thinks a prescription is needed. This might happen, for example, if a woman has come to the centre because she is embarrassed about talking to her doctor about having thrush.

The centre has been publicised on television, with free 20-second Public Service announcements on HTV West. Local radio broadcasts have also proved productive. Leaflets are distributed via the Women's Institute, the Townswomen's Guild, libraries, citizens advice bureaux and the Samaritans. Members of the committee give talks to womens' groups around the county; their audiences have been extremely supportive. Committee members have also spoken at a weekly meeting for health visitors, who were very sympathetic. Publicity to doctors has been happening through word of mouth; it was decided that it might have seemed defensive to write round beforehand. All GPs would in any case have seen the initial advertisement for a doctor for the centre, circulated via the Family Practitioner Committee. Some sympathetic GPs have been making referrals. The centre's supporters are also hoping to talk to GP trainees, who are often receptive to new ideas.

Are the objectives being achieved?

The volunteers who help at the centre clearly feel that their work is proving to be necessary; as one helper, Grace, said 'how can they say the service is already provided – otherwise how would we have so many here?' Women ranging in age from under 16 to 80 have come from miles around, as the centre's reputation spreads by word of mouth. Jenny points out that 'Sometimes they come from 30 miles away – they must be desperate. When they've seen the doctor we ask "was it worth the journey?" and they always say thankfully "Yes!" Sometimes people stuff £5 notes into the donation box.' The centre provides a free service; donations are entirely voluntary. Several committee members feel that some women would be put off if a charge was made.

Women come with very different problems: sometimes a whole afternoon is devoted to smear tests, sometimes a woman comes feeling suicidal. The main age range is from 30 to 60. Often people want information about gynaecological matters, which their doctor has not explained properly. The centre's records show that questions about the menopause (10 per cent of clients), requests for cervical smears (11 per cent), and breast examinations (10 per cent), figure prominently. About 30 per cent of clients come with emotional worries. Many problems stem from a combination of reasons: for example, if a woman is told she has to have a hysterectomy and is not given proper information about it, an emotional problem can follow.

The women who come to the centre often say that they appreciate the welcoming atmosphere, and the chance to talk to a sympathetic woman doctor. One woman said, 'It's taken me four weeks to pluck up the courage to come – it's a lot better than I expected! I've just lost my husband and the doctor said, well you always get these aches and pains when you're bereaved.' When she came out after seeing the doctor she looked very relieved: 'It's such a load off my mind.' Grace, one of the helpers, remembers a woman coming in

61

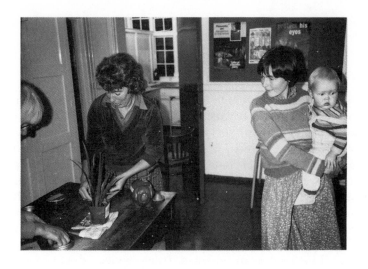

End of session at Taunton Well Woman Centre: volunteers tidy up and doctor collects her child

supported by her teenage daughter: 'Her hand was shaking so much she said "I can't have a cup of tea now". When she came out she was all smiles.'

The committee running the Well Woman Centre meets about once a month, and sees the idea of user control as very important. The committee selects the doctor who works at the centre. When the first doctor was being appointed, the committee disagreed with the District Community Physician, who was also present at the interviews. The DCP wanted someone with a lot of confidence, but the committee wanted someone more approachable because women might arrive very depressed. Committee members also questioned the interviewees on how they would feel about working with volunteers. The committee's choice was different from the DCP's, but he accepted the decision.

When the first doctor left, another round of interviews also produced a choice – one candidate had more experience in gynaecology and the other in psychiatry. The group decided that since the job was more concerned with counselling, psychiatric experience was probably more useful.

Lessons learned

There is a constant hope that the health authority will finally agree to give a grant to the Well Woman Centre. But official funding could bring complications with it. For example, would the steering committee still have control over important issues such as choosing the doctor to be employed? The centre's success depends on its being managed by users.

There are future plans for Well Woman Centres in other parts of Somerset. Groups are currently campaigning in Bridgwater and Yeovil. Another possibility is for a doctor to go round the villages, practising in different church halls, in which case the support of organisations like the rural community council would once again be needed in negotiating this new venture.

Whatever the exact nature of new developments, there is no doubt that the centre fulfils an important need. Most women have experienced difficulties with doctors at some point during their lives. Those who help at the centre, or attend as clients, come to realise that they are not alone in the feelings they have had. Women from different outlooks and backgrounds find a common cause in working together on the Well Woman Centre project.

5 *Neighbourhood Health Action*

Stockwell Health Project
Lady Margaret Hall Settlement, South London

Background

Within the structure of the National Health Service, there is
little provision for consumers to have a say in the planning of
their health care. Community health councils, set up in 1974
as 'watchdogs' on behalf of the public, can put forward
opinions about any plans they receive, but their views will
not necessarily be taken into account. Is it possible to create
new channels of communication between planners and those
who actually use the services concerned? Although a community health project may have wider goals than change in
the NHS, discussion of a particular local health service may
be a good place to start.

Stockwell is an inner city area in south London, contain-
ing several large old housing estates, tower blocks and some
newer estates. There are high numbers of elderly people,
unemployed people and single parents, many of whom have
stressful lives and need to use services frequently.

In 1979, after years of delay, a new health centre was
finally scheduled to be built in the area. A group of residents,
local workers, and Community Health Council representatives met to discuss the plans. The meetings began under the
auspices of the Stockwell and Vauxhall Neighbourhood
Council, a voluntary group funded by Lambeth Council. Its
brief is to involve residents in discussing issues which affect
their locality.

The Stockwell and Vauxhall Neighbourhood Health
Group encouraged people to say what they wanted from the
health centre. Pensioners' groups, parents' groups and
others had positive suggestions for the services they would

65

like to see provided. There was clearly an interest in health issues.

The health group successfully sought funding to establish a community health project with a paid worker. The first meeting of Stockwell Health Project (SHP) took place in September 1980. Since then, there have been three successive workers: Marcelle Rudolph, Pat Gonsalves and Janet Hibbert, and two social work students did placements with the project: Tricia Swaby and Susie Mackie. The workers have been based at Lady Margaret Hall Settlement in Stockwell, where administrative work can be done with secretarial support.

Funding

Initially, the worker's salary was provided jointly by the King Edward's Hospital Fund for London (the King's Fund) and the Special Trustees of St Thomas' Hospital. The funding application was sponsored by Lady Margaret Hall Settlement, an established voluntary organisation which had housed community projects for many years. After the first two years, further funding was obtained from Inner City Partnership via West Lambeth Health Authority. The money was granted for a three-year period, and was then extended for a further year.

Objectives

The health project's aim is to help local residents to take an active interest in their own health. It is seen as vital to involve local black and working-class women in the project's work.

The project wishes to act as a source of information so that people can make the best use of health services. A key objective is to encourage people to meet, on a group or individual basis, to discuss health issues: to explore how health problems are linked with other difficulties in their lives, and to gain information and support from each other so that they can make changes in their situation.

Through work such as the health centre project, it is hoped to encourage people to communicate their ideas to the authorities, and to participate in the management of their own health care.

The project is aware of the need to increase people's confidence, by making sure that all members are involved in discussions and decision-making.

Activities

Mawbey Brough Health Centre project

The report by Stockwell and Vauxhall Neighbourhood Council Health Group, *Mawbey Brough – A Health Centre for the Community?* (January 1980) specified what would be needed in the new health centre. For example, many local women wanted an open-door clinic where they could take their children to a nurse for first-aid treatment, to avoid having to go to the hospital casualty department for minor accidents. The Neighbourhood Council pensioners' group suggested that meetings or self-help groups could be arranged at the health centre, on topics such as arthritis and keep-fit. Youth workers were keen to see a counselling and information service on contraception, abortion and sexually transmitted infections.

Other needs identified included: an open-door counselling service for all sections of the community; opticians', dentists', and chiropodists' services available to everyone; and a post for a community health worker who could link the health centre with its users.

The report pointed out that doctors should be encouraged to come into the health centre and practise as a team. Finally, the health group wanted direct community involvement on the managing body of the health centre, and proposed joining with representatives of the health authority to form a steering group whilst the centre was being planned and built.

The health group held public meetings on the plans for the health centre, discussing the building design in detail. The group met with members of the health authority's District Management Team, with Lambeth Council architects, and with the NHS project group responsible for the health centre, to put across local people's views. The district community physician also met with the health group and offered support.

Dissatisfied with the council architects' design for the health centre, the health group asked Matrix, a group of women architects, to draw up some alternatives. Three possible designs were produced, based on the needs expressed by local people. The design finally chosen included a community café as the central point, meeting space for community groups and areas of privacy where people could wait to see health workers or counsellors.

The District Management Team, however, were unwilling to revise the original design, saying that this would cause delays in the building work and might lead to the project being cancelled altogether. However, they were impressed by the health group's design, and said that they hoped to incorporate some features of it into the final product.

The DMT also agreed that a joint group should be set up to make recommendations about the health centre's operation. In December 1980, representatives from the health group and the DMT started to discuss the aims and functions of such a 'project group'. By March 1981, it had been agreed that the Mawbey Brough Health Centre Project Group would recommend which services should be provided at the centre, how they should be provided, and how community representatives should be involved in the centre's management. The project group would comprise five of the district's more senior officers, a member of the Planning Department, six members of the Stockwell Health Project, and Community Health Council representatives.

The project group proceeded to discuss the importance of preventive health care, the particular health needs of different sections of the community, and how more GPs could be appointed in the area. The project group decided that all the services previously requested by community organisations should be provided. In a report to the DMT, they also recommended that a multi-ethnic group of staff should be appointed, including a woman doctor for Asian women, that there should be information in several languages and an ethnic minorities community worker.

Mawbey Brough Health Centre was finished in 1984, but

the final design has incorporated very few of Stockwell Health Project's suggestions. The district health authority has offered community representatives 'consultative' status only on the management committee.

The Mawbey Brough Health Centre work has been the only part of Stockwell Health Project to gain official recognition within the NHS. However, many of those involved in the project feel that other kinds of work have been more important, as described below.

Anti-racist health work

The project considers that this should be a basic every-day part of any community health work. Stockwell Health Project has helped to get funding for a Bengali health project, an Asian woman community health worker, and a community worker for racial minorities in the area. One of SHP's proposals for Mawbey Brough Health Centre was that there should be a black community health worker on the staff. Work has also been done with other interested organisations to try to set up special ante-natal English classes for Portuguese women, and a community translation project.

Health groups

An important focus of Stockwell Health Project's work has been women's health support groups, which have gone beyond a discussion of health service provision and taken a holistic approach to health. Two groups have run on a long-term basis with the support of project workers.

Pat Gonsalves helped a mother and toddler group on Lansdowne Green Estate to arrange their own course on children's health. Topics in the 12-week programme included asthma, head lice, hyper-active children, and how to answer young children's questions about sex. The course proved successful, and women became interested in looking at their own health. Another 12 sessions were arranged, funded by the local adult education institute. Subjects included migraine, cancer, women's legal rights and natural medicine. There was so much information to cover that the programme went on for five months.

69

Angela, who has been a member of the group from the beginning, found the group particularly helpful when she had to have an operation:

> I had support to look after the children while I was in hospital. I had books to read, and I decided what I thought about my treatment. If I hadn't had the information I would just have accepted what they said. After I'd had the operation I could talk about it in the group.

The group also helped Angela to prepare a list of questions to ask at the hospital.

A session with the community dietitian on food raised a lot of interest. Some members of the group formed a 'Get-Slim Get Well' club. They publicised the club via leaflets put in shops and launderettes, and handed out at school gates. Again, a tutor was provided by the adult education institute. The group grew to about 12 women, and met for several months. Members discussed the pressures on women to slim: as one person said of the group at the time, 'There is no one bullying you or making you feel ashamed if you've gained a pound or two. We hope to reach a weight that is our ideal and not what we are supposed to be.' Every week, the group cooked a good healthy lunch, with different people bringing recipes from their own countries. The club decided to collect the recipes in a *Healthy Food* pamphlet which could be sold to raise funds.

Women from Lansdowne Green, along with other groups, went to a women's Health Fair in Scotland in 1983. They remember that 'we took all the kids and it was nice to get away'.

Recently, the group has done some 'fun things', doing each other's hair and make-up, going to the sauna, going shopping together. They found that these activities gave them 'a lift'. As one women said, 'How much time a week do you spend on yourself? It's great to get out without the kids sometimes.'

Another women's health group is based at Sherborne House Drop-in Centre. This group originally began on the Lambeth Health Bus, and moved into the drop-in centre with the help of Stockwell Health Project worker Pat Gonsalves.

The group made a list of what everybody wanted to talk about, and soon had to fix a time-limit of three weeks per topic because discussions went on for so long. Subjects included sexuality, rape, cancer, doctors, racism and prostitution. As Sally says, 'We never said anything's not relevant, because if it's affecting you it's affecting your health.'

The method used to discuss each topic was to pool everyone's knowledge. For example, when discussing alternative medicine, one member could talk about having been to an osteopath, another to an acupuncturist, and so on. Between them, the group members discovered a wealth of information. Women gave each other advice: Maureen points out that 'people have had the same experiences and it's good to find out how others coped'. Pat Gonsalves arranged for health books to be borrowed from the library, and this back-up information was found to be of great help.

The trust built up in the group was essential. People could speak openly because it had been agreed that nobody would betray confidences outside the group. Sometimes a whole session was given over to somebody's personal problem if the need was urgent.

Sally found the group a relief: 'It makes you feel you're not just an anxious mother. My two children had whooping-cough and it wasn't diagnosed ... so many things came out about doctors.' Sonia used to suffer from anxiety attacks which, through the group, she realised were due to stress: 'The doctor said "go home and grow up". I thought I was having heart attacks.'

The group arranged a week's holiday for 25 adults and 34 children, which was a great success. They have also visited health groups in other areas to exchange ideas and information.

Stress group

The problem of women feeling under stress, and sometimes being dependent on tranquillisers, has come up in the Stockwell Health Project's work. In June 1983, Pat Gonsalves started a 'Women and Stress' group, drawing in women from the existing health groups who had expressed

71

interest. The format was partly to talk about feelings, and partly to do massage and relaxation work, with a tutor funded by Morley College.

At the first meeting, about twenty women were present. The group discovered that it was common for women to focus on other people's needs and pay little attention to themselves. Members sometimes made a 'contract' with the group, for example to do something they enjoyed before the next week's meeting. Several women found this very satisfying.

After meeting for over a year, the group got very small, and ended temporarily. Janet Hibbert, the Stockwell Health Project worker, decided to restart the group in March 1985. The new group is called 'Women Talking'. Janet didn't want the publicity to be too depressing, 'otherwise stress can feel like something you can't get out of, whereas in fact there *are* highlights in life'. She hopes that women will bring their strengths to the group: 'Whatever we've been through we have survived, and we can build on that.'

Other health work

Other groups have dealt with specific topics: pre-menstrual tension, for example, and menopause. These groups have tended to have a brief life span: the broader approach of the general health groups seems to have been more inspiring, enabling women to discuss all aspects of well-being. The project has helped to generate a number of other activities: for example, arranging a new venue for a baby clinic by negotiating with a tenants' association to use a community flat; bringing together workers concerned with young people's health, who decided to produce a directory of local contraceptive services; and compiling a directory of health-related services in Stockwell, which was done by Tricia Swaby, one of the social work students on placement.

Two health events were organised in the first two years. One was a play on health issues, performed in the premises of a local school. Another was a health day, held in a youth club building and attended by about two hundred local people. Many organisations and self-help groups had stalls, and there were films, speakers and a free health lunch.

Arriving as the new worker in September 1984, Janet decided to offer six-week courses on health topics to interested community groups. The first was run in a day centre for the elderly, and covered safety in the home, diabetes, hypothermia, bereavement and welfare rights. Those attending enjoyed the course, 'especially finding out that they were entitled to more benefits!'

Janet organised another course at Ifeoma, a residential mother and baby home for young black women. Here the topics included 'our lives as black women', relationships with others, violence, contraception and a visit to a black women's health group.

Other groups who may be interested in a health course

73

include the Family Support Service, Lambeth Latchkey Service and a local secondary school.

Are the objectives being achieved?

Since 1979, a number of people in the Stockwell area, mainly women, have been consistently involved in discussing health matters, through groups and events initiated by the Stockwell Health Project. By the end of the first three years, 1,196 women had been in contact with the project; the form of contact ranged from asking for a particular item of information at an event to joining a health group. At one point, 250 women were involved in the various groups. To ensure that all women feel able to attend the health groups, child care is always provided and publicity is written to welcome both black and white women. All groups have been racially mixed.

The project has made health information more widely available via literature such as the directory of contraceptive services and the directory of health-related services, and via public meetings about the Mawbey Brough Health Centre, and events such as the 1982 Health Day.

A number of health groups have met for varying periods of time. All have enabled the participants to relate health problems to other issues: for example, bad housing conditions, lack of healthy food or difficulties with doctors. Group members speak appreciatively of the practical knowledge they have gained, and give numerous examples of being able to express their views more confidently to health workers. Sonia from the Sherborne House group points out that 'groups are good for people. A lot of women are isolated. I now have support outside the group as well as in, which I didn't have before.' There is a sense of community amongst the women who have attended health groups. They help each other in practical ways, such as babysitting or decorating a new flat.

This support has affected members' lives in other significant ways. Sally thinks that 'It's helped us to find our identity.' The project's goal has been to use health groups as a springboard to other activities. Women have stayed in the

74

groups for as long as is useful to them, and then gone on to further education, part-time jobs, or training courses such as a three-year course in painting and decorating. Maureen began youth work: 'With the group I realised I wasn't the only one that felt chained ... you want something more out of life.'

Those involved in the Mawbey Brough Health Centre project found it difficult to deal with health service bureaucracy. However, Stockwell Health Project members continued to press for their opinions to be taken into account. Group members became more confident about expressing their views at official meetings. After the first year of work in the joint project group, SHP representatives thought that the health service members had in fact become more sympathetic to ideas coming from the community side.

Although the specific aims of the SHP for the health centre have not been achieved, the more general aim of organising local people to voice their opinions on health care has been realised. It is rare to have set up a working group where members of a local community meet directly with health service officials. It is equally unusual for a community group to propose its own design for a health service building and to get that design seriously considered. The Stockwell Health Project representatives on the working group kept in constant touch with local health groups, obtaining their views about how negotiations should proceed.

SHP asked for the help of local councillors when difficulties over the lease threatened to stop the building of the health centre. The fact that a community group was constantly watching over the project may have been crucial at this point.

SHP fosters community participation within its own organisation. The decision-making body is the Stockwell Health Project group, which is made up entirely of local black and working-class women. Therefore the project is actually being run by people from the local community. Offices rotate in order to give everyone the chance to develop new skills.

Lessons learned

Mawbey Brough Health Centre work

This work might have been more fruitful if SHP had been involved from the beginning, before the initial design was drawn up. When the recommendations of the joint project group were disregarded, SHP decided in principle to withdraw from involvement in the health centre.

No GPs have yet been attracted to work in the health centre, and community participation has been low. Will the health authority come to recognise that if SHP's advice had been taken into account, the health centre could have been much more successful?

SHP received TV and newspaper coverage during the health centre campaign. Requests for information have been coming in from other projects around the country. SHP has made people aware that it is possible to become involved in a health authority's planning process. The work done on Mawbey Brough Health Centre may help projects elsewhere to be more successful. It has also provided an excellent practical focus through which to draw people into the wider community health work of SHP.

Health groups

Both women's health groups are now uncertain as to how to progress. Women who have attended for some time feel that they have run out of topics to discuss. Do the groups still need the constant help of the community health worker, or are they ready to be self-sufficient? Group members commented on the advantages of weekly contact with the worker: 'to bring in new ideas'; 'to push us in the right direction'; 'to help us fill in forms for funding'.

Janet feels that the groups should be able to take the initiative themselves now. They may want to remain as a support group for members, but in that case, should the community health worker move on to start work on new projects? Could the current women's health groups build on the wealth of information they have obtained, by addressing other groups on health subjects? There is a danger that, as Janet says, 'it's women working for nothing again'. She is investigating the possibility of the groups being paid for giving talks, and for writing information sheets on health.

The need for more workers

The community health workers at Stockwell Health Project have always had a huge workload. Janet is convinced that one post is not enough, and points out that most other community health projects have more workers. 'If you really are about change and preventive care, you need more back-up.'

She also feels the need for someone with whom she can discuss issues such as: how can her time best be used? Is her role to run groups, or just to start them up by linking people together? Energy can easily be spread too thin, and Janet is wary of starting things she cannot prolong.

Is it better to start discussion groups, or campaigning groups, or both? Janet sees campaigns against cuts in the health service as very important. To do campaigning work effectively, she would like to have back-up from people who are familiar with the workings of local government and the NHS.

Community health work can take a long time to show results, but Janet is hopeful about the future. 'Five years will never be enough to see a big change in people's attitudes, and there is a lot of hard work to be done. But I feel optimistic that local people *are* involved and will become more independent.'

6 *Housing*

'The Blocks are No Place For Children' Campaign
Bristol Settlement

Background

The tower blocks which loom over Bristol Settlement date
from the 1950s and 1960s. Throughout Britain at this time,
terraced houses were demolished to build what was thought
to be 'more advanced' housing. Tenants of the new high-rise
flats rapidly discovered problems, including dampness and
condensation, inadequate heating, feelings of isolation, and
the practical difficulties of negotiating stairs and lifts. The
effects on health were alarming. Residents in the Barton Hill
tower blocks have tried to deal with their housing problems
by organising tenants' groups.

In 1981, the Community Development Unit was set up
within Bristol Settlement to undertake community work in
the neighbourhood, to be a base for social work students on
placement, and to do relevant local research. In April 1982,
Sarah Cemlyn, who supervised the students, arranged to
meet the chairman and secretary of the residents' association. She asked them if there was any work they might like a
student to undertake.

> We stood in the secretary's flat and looked out at another
> block, and we kept seeing nappies drying. She said 'They're
> not supposed to house children here but they keep moving
> them in.'

The first student to become involved checked the council's policy. It was indeed that children under 14 should not
be housed in high-rise flats. He checked the registers at local
playgroups and nursery schools to get an idea of the number
of children actually living in the blocks. When he went to

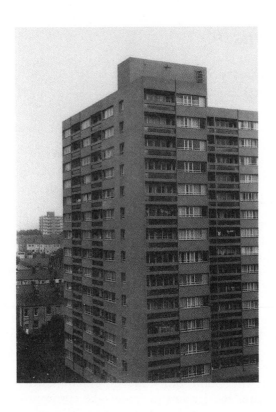

Block of high-rise flats, Barton Hill, Bristol.
Credit: Blocks Campaign

interview families with children resident there, he found them angry about their situation.

Parents were finding it stressful to live without nearby playspace for their children. The only outside space was the balconies, which were completely unprotected; accidents could have been fatal. One women had found her child sitting on the balcony on the thirteenth floor. Lifts constantly broke down, which meant that children and shopping had to be carried upstairs, a physically exhausting task. Finally, damp was causing or aggravating children's illnesses such as bronchitis.

The interviewing produced such a response that the two students now working on the issue prepared and delivered a leaflet, explaining the situation and suggesting a meeting. When the meeting took place, in November 1982, there was a strong feeling that action was needed. A campaign was set up, called 'The Blocks Are No Place For Children'. The 13 people present decided to form a committee.

> All kids who live in tower blocks are restricted kids, and all their mothers are under pressure ... We believe that kids should grow up looking up at birds and trees and not looking down on them.
>
> (John Hall, member of the Blocks Campaign)

Funding and resources

The Community Development Unit began in 1981 with few resources. Funding for Sarah Cemlyn's part-time post as student supervisor was paid for out of student placement funds. From February 1982, the Community Enterprise Programme of the Manpower Services Commission gave funding for a neighbourhood worker, Alison Gilchrist, for one year. Alison's time was mainly occupied by supporting the community newspaper, the *Feeder*. In September 1983, the Settlement obtained Voluntary Project Programme funding for its outreach work, and Alison was reappointed for another year. This time she was able to concentrate on supporting the Blocks Campaign. At this point the Community Development Unit's name changed to the Community Development Project; thus it is referred to here as the CDU/CDP.

The Blocks Campaign has always been independent from the Settlement, with support from the CDU/CDP workers and students. From October 1982 to the end of March 1983, there were always two students working with the Campaign. At times when there have been no student placements and no funds for workers, Sarah Cemlyn has had to keep the CDU/CDP going and help the Blocks group where possible.

Objectives

The Blocks Campaign has had two main concerns: to enable families with children already living in high-rise flats to move to low-rise accommodation (preferably with a garden),

81

and to prevent the council from housing more children in the blocks.

In backing the group, the CDU/CDP has been careful to follow its own principle: 'to help local people working collectively to make improvements in the neighbourhood and to increase their control over decisions affecting their lives'. The unit did not intend to lead the campaign, but to provide appropriate resources of information and energy. Students and workers always considered that the way of working adopted by the group, involving all members and helping them to become more confident, was just as important as the practical results achieved.

Activities

With eight or nine people consistently involved in the group, the Blocks Campaign made rapid progress. Most of those in the group had children. One couple's children had already grown up and left home, but the couple felt strongly that the difficulties they had experienced should not have to be faced by others. Meetings took place in members' flats or at the Settlement (making use of the crèche facilities there).

Previous tenants' groups had had a more sober style, meeting with the council to pass on complaints. The Blocks group were militant from the start. Early in 1983, a giant banner with the campaign slogan printed on it was hung from the thirteenth floor of one of the blocks. Shortly afterwards, a huge Valentine card was delivered to the chairman of the housing committee, with a 1,000-signature petition demanding action. These events attracted a lot of attention from the local media, with front-page coverage exposing the harshness and indifference of the council and radio and TV interviews.

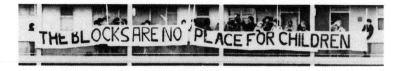

Banner with campaign slogan hung from tower block balcony. *Credit: Blocks Campaign*

The council required the campaign to produce evidence about the numbers of children actually housed in the blocks, before officials would take any action. The group therefore did a door-to-door survey of the three blocks where the majority of children were living. At the same time, they gathered more details about the difficulties of living in the flats with children, and found that many people lacked correct information about the workings of the transfer system.

The campaign asked the council to give extra points to families with children under 14. In February 1983, the council finally agreed to do so, which enabled some families to rise to the top of the transfer list and move out. The apparent victory was soon found to be a hollow one. Families with children were still being moved into the blocks, despite the council's reaffirmation of its policy, and these new families were *not* being given the increased points.

The campaign wrote to all members of the housing committee to complain about this situation. In February 1984, the director of housing wrote to the group to say that the Housing Department wanted to give people a choice about where they lived, rather than being 'paternalistic'. The Blocks group pointed out that people could not make real choices if they were not given enough information. Families were not being told about the drawbacks of living in the flats, nor about the way the points system worked.

Finally, the group met with the Special Projects officers from the Housing Department, to write a leaflet to be given to all families with children who were offered flats in the blocks. The leaflet suggested that people should think carefully before deciding whether to accept the council's offer or wait longer for other accommodation. It described in detail – from a parent's point of view – what it was like to live in the blocks with children, covering points such as lack of play facilities, dangerous balconies, the dependence on lifts and feelings of isolation.

The campaign was also responsible for opening a community room in one of the blocks, for the use of a parent and toddler group. The Blocks group pressured the council to give a grant of £2,500 to make the premises suitable. The parent and toddler group is now functioning independently of the Blocks group.

During the campaign, publicity has appeared in the *Feeder*, a newspaper produced by a local group using the facilities and support of the CDU/CDP. Tim Bickell, a volunteer who works on the *Feeder*, points out the essential difference between a community newspaper and the rest of the media: 'The ordinary media take up a campaign like this at peak moments, then drop it like a hot brick when it goes off the boil.' The *Feeder* reported the campaign consistently and accurately, often giving front-page coverage to articles which might have been relegated to a corner in another newspaper.

Have the objectives been achieved?

Members of the Blocks Campaign feel that they are nearly at the end of their road. Some families with children have already been moved to low-rise accommodation. The parent and toddler group helps to improve life for families still living in the flats, although the campaign has made it clear that these families must eventually be rehoused. Parents being offered a high-rise flat will now receive the campaign's information leaflet, so fewer are likely to move in. Bristol City Council is restructuring its points and allocation system and is taking into consideration the representations of the Blocks Campaign. The remaining members of the group are already putting their energies into new community activities, such as a tenants' group on the estate, the Barton Hill Action Group.

Sarah Cemlyn thinks that the students and workers have accurately followed the CDU/CDP's guidelines for community work. 'People operate in very different ways and community workers have to adapt to that. The style of the Blocks Campaign has been direct and militant.' Students and workers have encouraged the group to learn new skills: for example, by working with group members to write official letters, until campaigners could do this alone, and could teach others. In preparation for a meeting with the director of housing, the group did a role-play of the meeting, and were able to speak more confidently when the meeting took place. The students and workers have also made sure that the group was in contact with sympathetic people in organisations like the local CVS and Shelter, so that the campaign had its own information sources.

Involvement in the campaign has had beneficial effects on many members. One woman described the improvement in her mental health:

> Before I became involved with the campaign I was very depressed and isolated. The doctor had given me tablets to combat the depression, but all they did was make me very tired . . . Just before I become involved with the campaign I ran out of tablets . . . A few months passed and I realised I felt better and didn't have time to be depressed and I certainly was no longer isolated. The campaign was a better medicine than drugs.

Others also found new strengths, or rediscovered their abilities. One woman had been in the group for three months before she even had the courage to say that she could type, yet she was the person who later took on the demanding task of speaking at a Trades Council meeting. Another woman, again after quite a while, disclosed that she had graphic talent, and became involved in the production of the *Feeder*.

Tim Bickell saw the change in those who worked on the newspaper. At one point, volunteers from the campaign devoted their energies to helping the paper through a difficult period. 'It gave the Blocks Campaign people a chance to discover talents and skills they already had . . . I see people now who've got a lot more confidence in themselves.'

Lessons to be learned

Collective work has not always been easy. The group became aware of the need to share tasks, otherwise the load could fall on a few people and be exhausting.

Some members of the group have been rehoused (in fact the council has a tendency to rehouse activists first), which could have threatened the group's cohesion, or set up a conflict with those who were staying in the blocks. However, two of those who have left the flats continued to work with the campaign for a while, even though it meant a long journey with small children.

Occasionally there have been misunderstandings with other tenants. At one point the Tenants' Action Group thought that the Blocks Group was giving the flats a bad name. The campaign had to make it clear that the issue they were complaining about was that the blocks were not a good place for children. On another occasion, it was discovered that the playroom was going to be sited in a block where residents had not been consulted. The siting was moved to another block where adequate consultation *was* carried out.

One problem for the CDU/CDP throughout has been its lack of consistent funding. It has been hard to maintain continuity in supporting the campaign, with students only coming for three- or six-month placements, and workers often having to concentrate on other projects.

It is a tribute to the energy and persistence of the Blocks group that they have managed to keep going despite all difficulties. For local people, the campaign has obviously touched on a very real concern of theirs. As the campaign members go on to new activities, their experience in organising will be of great benefit to others.

7 *Food*

Crumbles Community Café
Bristol Settlement

Background

A high-fibre, low-fat diet is now recognised to be a basic requirement for good health. However, it can be hard to find shops or cafés which provide this kind of food.

The Barton Hill Youth Project began over five years ago, based at Bristol Settlement. The project's work included the training of unemployed young people in catering. It was decided to run a wholefood café on the premises, to give the trainees work experience. The café could also contribute to the general welfare of settlement users, since having a sustaining meal at lunchtime can help people to stay healthy and work through the day.

Funding and resources

Barton Hill Youth Project is a Youth Training Scheme, funded by the Manpower Services Commission, which pays salaries to the four staff and weekly allowances to the trainees. Staff include the co-ordinator, Erzsi Lyne de Ver, and the catering supervisor, Joan Phelan. These two are responsible for the work being done in the café, along with Carolyn Coupland, who works three days a week with her wages paid from café profits.

Objectives

The café aims to provide healthy food for settlement users and the Barton Hill community. Through their work in the café, the catering trainees are intended to gain experience of preparing and cooking food, dealing with stock control and relating to the public. Because Crumbles is a wholefood café, they can also learn about good nutrition, and find out how to use ingredients and cooking methods which are new to them. The café thus has the potential to meet a number of needs simultaneously.

Activities

Joan Phelan and Carolyn Coupland work with four trainees, keeping the café open for lunch and snacks every day except Friday. Popular dishes which are regularly on offer include soups, vegetable pie, cheese and leek pie, chili con carne, vegetarian lasagne, whole wheat pizza and spaghetti bean bake. Ingredients are usually vegetarian but sometimes include meat. The idea is to provide wholesome food which is easy to eat.

The trainees look for recipes in cookbooks such as *The Bean Book* and *The Vegetarian Epicure*; Joan and Carolyn check that the suggestions are appropriate for use in the café. Selected recipes are then written up by the trainees in the café's own loose-leaf cookbook. Sometimes the names are changed to make them sound more attractive: the dish of 'crumble' is called 'vegetables with crunchy cheese topping' instead.

On Friday, when the café is closed, the trainees have a chance to try out new recipes and practise cookery skills.

Are the objectives being achieved?

Crumbles provides a useful meeting place for workers and volunteers at the settlement. One member of staff pointed out that with everyone so heavily involved in their own projects, the café might be the only place where people could meet in a relaxed way, to discuss work or for social reasons.

The café food is enjoyed by many of the staff. On a day when it was unexpectedly closed, several people were at a loss to find anywhere else for lunch locally, and mutters were heard of 'Where's my lentil soup?' Volunteers rely particularly on the cheap prices in the café, since they receive a food allowance of only 50p a day.

Customers show their appreciation by asking for recipes,

and wanting to know 'Who made the soup today?' The cakes are a special favourite. Joan admits that 'cakes are really my weakness – I think a piece of cake now and then is OK if everything else you eat is healthy. I use half the amount of sugar in the recipes.' Cakes may be the first attraction for many customers, encouraging them to come in and use the café. Hopefully they will gradually start to try the less familiar items on the menu.

Perhaps the biggest changes in eating habits are seen amongst the trainees themselves. Joan finds it very satisfying to see their attitudes change from 'What's that? I'm not eating that!' to a genuine enjoyment of wholefoods. Once they start to taste and make the new dishes, their prejudices are overcome. Instead of eating chips and beefburgers, they often start to cook flans and vegetables at home, thus introducing their families to wholefoods, too. One trainee moved to her own flat and took a selection of the café recipes with her. Another visited a café where a friend worked, and later told Joan that the smell of grease was terrible. 'She said that she'd hate to have to work somewhere like that, and she'd only become aware of this since she started to work with me.'

Another pleasing result of Joan's work is that most of her trainees do get jobs in catering. 'Even if they're low-paid, at least it's a start.' This is quite unusual in the context of Youth Training Schemes.

Lessons learned

Some difficulties have arisen from the nature of the youth project. The trainees sometimes feel resentful about working hard for so little pay. There is often a conflict between trying to provide the best training for the young people, and trying to stay open to the community for as many hours as possible.

The café is not widely used by people from Barton Hill, other than those who already come into the settlement. The café's entrance is rather hidden away, and perhaps some people do not realise that it is open to everyone. A board may be set up outside, showing the daily menu and prices.

Another problem may prove more taxing to solve. Some

users of the café, both settlement workers and members of groups meeting at the settlement, have criticised the food provided. Erzsi, the co-ordinator of the youth project, thinks that long-term eating habits are hard to change, and change certainly cannot be forced. She wonders whether community workers, who are often under a lot of pressure, tend not to look after their own needs. With smoking, for example, 'they need their fifty cigarettes a day and they're reluctant to give them up and look at their own health'. A similar 'resistance to health consciousness' may occur over nutrition. Erzsi remembers her own views in the past: 'When I heard people talk about health, I used to think "how boring".' She recognises that it's very easy to sound evangelical, which does not make people feel like listening.

Members of the community groups who use the settlement are often battling against difficult living conditions. They may not be able to concentrate on changing their eating habits. Erzsi finds examples of this amongst the trainees themselves. All are going through the transition from school to adult life, which in itself can be a stressful time. They may have family problems, but do not have enough money to leave home. They have no previous experience of healthy eating patterns, and those not actually working in the café are not so interested in trying new foods.

One trainee had Type A infectious hepatitis: her doctor did not tell her she needed a high-protein/low-fat diet, with plenty of vitamins. Erzsi knew such a diet was important, but 'It was no good me just saying "you need this".' Another trainee became pregnant, and was used to smoking, staying up late, and not eating well: 'It's hard to explain that childbirth might be more difficult or she might have an unhealthy baby.'

However, would the right course be to provide 'what local people want', as suggested recently by some members of the settlement Executive Committee? The committee had received a complaint from members of the parents' group which meets at the settlement, saying that they had to take their children home at lunchtime because they wouldn't eat the café food.

Eating habits obviously can change, and people from very

different backgrounds can enjoy wholefoods, as shown by the experiences of the trainees working in the café. Perhaps the key factors are that the trainees have the chance to taste foods which look strange to them (without having to pay!), that in the process of cooking the dishes they become familiar with the ingredients and no longer mistrust the end result, and that they find out why 'junk foods' are bad for them.

How could some of these experiences be introduced to a wider audience? Erzsi and Joan are considering possible new ventures. Perhaps a 'taste-in' could be arranged at the café, to which groups using the settlement could be invited. Trainees in other sectors of the youth project could become involved in preparing for this event too, with each person making one dish. The cooks could go round and talk to the people trying out their dishes. The taste-in could be free, and reduced-price lunches could be advertised as a follow-up. Many people do not think of going to eat lunch in a café, since they do not feel able to spend much money on themselves.

Another possibility might be to invite groups using the settlement to cook in the café's kitchen, bringing their own recipes. They could learn to cook something that they *do* like from the menu; the young mothers' group, for example, appreciate the cakes. They might then want to try out other dishes which seem less familiar. The main difficulty is that the café is in constant use during the day, and Joan's time is fully taken up with the trainees. Joan is keen to offer an evening cookery class, although this might attract a different group of people, rather than the regular settlement users. Perhaps talks on nutrition could be arranged during the day if groups were interested.

Finally, a lively way to provide education in the café itself could be the use of posters. Trainees could make these, perhaps using an example of 'junk food' such as a Swiss roll. Underneath a picture of the item, there could be a list of the additives it contains, which would probably surprise many people.

Nutrition education is needed to help people choose healthy food. When Joan gave a talk on nutrition to the parents' group, one woman, who wanted to eat healthily, was horrified to discover that brown bread is often white bread coloured with caramel. Joan points out that many working-class people don't have information about wholefoods, nor do they have the opportunity to obtain them: 'You can't buy wholemeal bread around here, only in trendy areas.' She wants to open up that choice to others.

Unhealthy food has particularly bad effects on people who are living in circumstances of stress and poverty. The café could give them a better chance.

8 *Self-Help Health Groups*

Self-Help Health Project for Northamptonshire
Northampton and County Council for Voluntary
Service and Northamptonshire Rural Community
Council

Background

Many self-help groups focus on health issues: often members are brought together by the need to talk about a common problem such as alcoholism or migraine, or the wish to learn more about bringing up children or about nutrition. Other groups, such as Age Concern, may have a more general brief, but definitely benefit people's health by helping them to live fuller and happier lives.

Teresa Middleton, development officer for volunteering at Northampton CVS, and Paul Carnell, of Northamptonshire RCC, both became aware of the potentially huge number of local self-help groups. Teresa gives some examples:

> A group to support people coming off tranquillisers asked me for practical help with publicity materials. A health visitor working with a self-help cancer group used to come and talk to me about her relationship with the group – it was hard for her to find that kind of back-up elsewhere. Then I'd get the occasional phone call asking things like "do you know of any groups for depression?"

There seemed to be a need to link together self-help groups in the county, and support their work. Teresa and Paul began to discuss these possibilities, and developed a programme for a Self-Help Health Project for Northamptonshire. Their initial paper described several key activities which could form the basis for the new project, such as a day workshop and the compilation of a local self-help index.

93

Funding and resources

Paul and Teresa have co-ordinated the Self-Help Health Project as part of their own jobs. Since the RCC and CVS have limited resources, other interested organisations such as the local community health councils and Health Education Department have been asked for help. Staff in these organisations have joined with the project, and have provided financial and administrative back-up.

Objectives

In the initial proposal, the project's purpose was explained as follows: to encourage the setting-up of self-help groups and to publicise their existence, both to people who might want to join, and to health and social services workers who could make referrals. It is clear that the project cannot itself set up groups: as Teresa says, 'It would be inappropriate to go out and start self-help groups – their very nature means they need to start themselves.' Instead, advice and resources can be offered to groups starting up, or to existing groups wishing to develop.

Activities

Paul is in contact with rural organisations such as the energetic Greens Norton 50 Plus Group, which runs educational activities and sessions for sports and keep-fit, led by people from the village. A retired GP is involved in 'health monitoring', seeing people regularly for long interviews. Paul comments that 'It's not at all the traditional club where things are arranged *for* elderly people by others; the whole feel of it is 'how can you join in?'

Another village, Kings Cliffe, may start something similar. Paul hopes to arrange an initial meeting between the Greens Norton group, an adult education organiser, and representatives from Age Concern and the Kings Cliffe Patient Participation Group. The latter is another active local self-help group: a committee of staff and patients from the Kings Cliffe practice meet monthly to discuss whether the practice is working well, and to organise local services

94

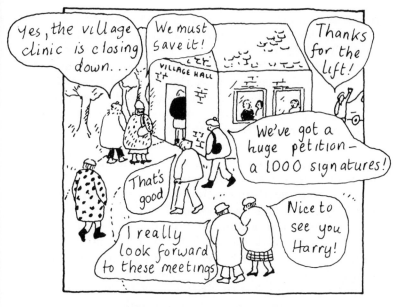

CHIRU Newsletter, winter 84/85

such as a voluntary car scheme. They have also lobbied to keep their local chiropody service.

Patient participation groups might work well in other areas too. Paul is also arranging discussion with medical practice workers, on the grounds that an RCC officer could prove a useful mediator between villagers and doctors' practices. Sometimes villagers have complaints about medical facilities, or doctors see the place provided for their branch surgery as inadequate. Such problems might be eased by bringing doctors and the parish council together to work out solutions.

Teresa keeps in touch with women's groups concerned with health. One Northampton women's group, Womanspace, wants to organise free pregnancy testing. Another group, attached to the Northampton Centre Against Unemployment, found that unemployed women are very interested in health issues. The centre ran a 14-week course on topics ranging from menopause to mental health, aiming to prepare women to become helpers at a Well Woman Centre. Teresa feels that maintaining contact between local women's

95

groups is important if a Well Woman Centre is to be sensitive to local need. Womanspace may soon be based in a council building; the centre could perhaps start there.

At an early stage, Teresa decided that it would be useful to visit similar projects, such as the Nottingham Self-Help Project, which now has its own premises. The existence of their starter pack for self-help groups made it unnecessary for the Northampton project to develop their own resource pack, which they had initially intended to do. Teresa was also able to build up a collection of books and other resources which self-help groups could refer to.

One of the project's first initiatives was a 'Health and Self-Help Day', to bring together local self-help groups, professionals, and other interested individuals, and encourage a county-wide network on self-help. In preparation for this event, Teresa and Paul visited as many groups as possible, and also talked to professionals. Publicity information was sent out to doctors, health visitors, social services and self-help groups, but most people came through personal contact and word of mouth.

The Day was held at Hunsbury Hill Centre, which is also the home of the RCC. The pleasant surroundings gave a relaxed feeling. Rooms were organised to produce a welcoming atmosphere, and an enjoyable wholefood lunch was provided. There was a small charge for the Day, with a higher fee for professionals.

Over 70 people attended, from a wide range of backgrounds. Teresa was nervous beforehand: 'It's rather like when you have a party and you think "How are all these people going to get on together?" – but they did! In fact, it was an incredible balance.'

Two speakers introduced the Day: Alison Watt from the Community Health Initiatives Resource Unit at NCVO, and the local district health education officer. Workshops followed on starting self-help groups, stress, women's health and patient participation groups. There was also plenty of time for people to talk to each other informally. The organisers had scoured local newspapers for articles on self-help groups, and displayed these, along with exhibitions and information brought along on the Day. Lists were put up so that people could add their name if they were interested in joining a group.

Another important task of the project has been the production of a Self-Help Index, a booklet listing local groups in Northamptonshire. Teresa, Paul and Jackie Walker (secretary of Northampton Community Health Council) did the research. Information was gathered from libraries, citizens advice bureaux, social services, volunteer bureaux and community centres. The Health Education Service designed the booklet and posters on the same theme. The production of the guide was financed by the CHC. The index was distributed to GPs surgeries (two copies each, one for the doctor and one for the receptionist), health visitors and workers in the social services.

The index was issued in a pilot form to test public reaction. The title does not use the word 'health', on the grounds that most people are not sure what a 'health group' is. An introductory section explains what self-help groups do, with quotes from members about their experiences. Groups are then listed under topic areas, without contact addresses. Readers are directed to phone their local CHC for further information about a particular group. This is because groups, and their addresses, change frequently. It is easier to update an index centrally than to keep producing new editions.

When people telephone for an address, they can also find out which group is most likely to be useful to them. For example, someone who asks about a group on depression might actually need a group on bereavement. People may feel uncertain about joining a group, and the CHC secretaries can encourage them to go along. If someone wants to start a new group, they can be referred to Teresa or Paul for support in doing so.

Paul has discovered that several voluntary car schemes, already in operation in rural areas, are willing to take people to self-help groups. This information will be passed on to the CHC secretaries, so that callers can be told about transport. Otherwise, people who are not mobile might assume that they could not attend a group.

The project proposal also mentioned the idea of a health

bus for rural areas, which would be both a mobile clinic and a health information centre. Paul is working with David Smith, adult education officer for Northamptonshire County Council, on a joint plan for a mobile resource centre. A double-decker bus could be used for a number of purposes simultaneously: a general advice service; an information point about job vacancies, volunteering opportunities and educational courses; and health-related activities, such as self-help groups, GP sessions, and a Well Woman Centre. Although this has generated quite a lot of interest, the prospects for funding are poor in the present climate.

Are the objectives being achieved?

Several of the ideas outlined in the project's initial proposal have been put into practice. The Health Day was an excellent start in linking self-help groups. Participants were keen to see a follow-up, especially to look at how groups could organise themselves. As a result, Paul and Teresa have arranged a week-end on group work and counselling for members of self-help groups. Funding from the Health Education Service has made it possible to charge only £5 per person. Paul has also obtained funds from the Development Commission for a volunteer, Lucy Kitto, to organise health days in rural centres around the country. The first will take place at Oundle where Lucy is working with a group of interested people to organise the day, with practical and financial support from the adult education organiser. By developing a strong local group, it is hoped that this will be a springboard for more activities in the area.

The response to the Self-Help Index has been encouraging, and the project plans to produce a second edition. Doctors and health visitors have asked for more copies, as has the School of Nursing. The CHC secretaries received over one hundred calls about the Index between August and November 1984. Kettering CHC noted that a number were about agoraphobia, and Northampton CHC noted several about bereavement.

Lessons learned

The project has achieved success by concentrating on activities which can be accomplished and evaluated. As Teresa says, 'Nothing has been rushed in this project; we take enough time to find out the best way to do something.'

The pilot edition of the Self-Help Index has generated ideas for future editions. Many people may not know what a 'self-help group' is; an alternative title could be 'groups to help you'. The CHC secretaries have had some problems with annoyed callers asking 'Why aren't there any addresses?' A new introduction will explain the reasons more clearly.

Larger enterprises such as a health bus need careful consideration. The idea has been greeted enthusiastically. Teresa has found that 'When you mention health buses people start to quiver with excitement – wholefood cookery on the move!' But careful thought has brought possible drawbacks to light. A mobile clinic can be cold in winter, there is nowhere for people to wait, and confidential discussions between patients and health workers can sometimes be overheard. As well as developing a proposal for a mobile unit, it is important to encourage schemes like that of the Kings Cliffe Patient Participation Group, in which elderly people from 12 villages are collected to go to a monthly clinic in a village hall, which is also a social event.

Teresa and Paul are well aware that the idea of 'self-help' is double-edged. Currently, there is a surge of interest in self-help. The DHSS is making available £10m for its programme 'Helping the Community to Care', of which £750,000 is earmarked for self-help groups. A local district health authority is encouraging self-help groups under its Strategic Plan, and may offer financial aid. According to Teresa, 'self-help can be used to undermine the statutory sector' if the promotion of self-help goes along with cuts in health and welfare services. She emphasizes that 'self-help is *not* a substitute for statutory services, it's complementary'.

Paul has the impression that 'self-help is providing something the NHS isn't at the moment – it releases energies from people which are bottled up because of the cult of professionalism'. If the NHS helped to set up self-help groups, would the control pass from lay people to professionals? The ideal role for professionals could be to work in a friendly capacity, to help with resources when a group is being set up, for example. Paul thinks that 'It's got to be an involvement in which you give the group more confidence and control, otherwise you perpetuate the relationships currently found within the NHS.'

At the Northamptonshire Health Day, there were more participants from self-help groups than professionals. This may have helped the professionals to join in more openly. Teresa comments that 'The atmosphere was conducive to being honest and informal, and the professionals began to say how *they* had been helped by self-help, what it meant to them on a personal level.'

The Northampton project is growing, and generating a lot of work for its organisers. Will it soon need its own worker? Is it a good idea to go further and create special centres for self-help groups, as has been done elsewhere? There are obvious advantages in this, but such places could become too large or too removed from contact with local groups, another danger of self-help becoming 'fashionable'.

The link-up between the CVS and RCC in Northamptonshire has proved very successful, enabling Teresa and Paul to pool their knowledge and develop work throughout the county. The project also demonstrates that, in order to work on health issues, it can be fruitful to link up with local Community Health Councils and Health Education Services. The scope for such an alliance is potentially very large, and a project on 'Self-Help and Health' has enormous possibilities.

9 *Community Care*

Manchester Alliance for Community Care
Manchester Council for Voluntary Service

Background

In the late 1980s, many people who have lived for years in state institutions because of chronic illness or disability will instead be placed 'in the community'. This process is part of the Government's plan to increase community care, and is bound to make considerable demands on the services provided by voluntary organisations. What are the likely results – positive and negative? What action can voluntary bodies take to make their voices heard on this issue?

In November 1981, the Manchester Council for Voluntary Service invited a number of interested people to meet and contribute their views on the Government's consultation document 'Care in the Community'. The response encouraged those present to convene the Manchester Alliance for Community Care (MACC). The individuals who came worked in organisations such as the CVS, Age Concern, the Spastics Society, Manchester Disability Forum, Central Manchester Community Health Council, MIND, MENCAP, and the Health Education Department. All shared the worry that, as a representative of the CHC puts it, 'people would just be dumped in the community,' without sufficient resources.

However, the group also examined the positive aspects of independent community care: the opportunities it could provide for independent living. They knew of ideas which seemed to work well. The Spastics Society, for instance, runs a 'Core and Cluster' scheme in Milton Keynes: a central building with staff and facilities serves a cluster of houses in the nearby area. Professionals in the 'core' building are on call, and emergency overnight beds are provided there. Another idea, being put into practice in Manchester, is for community service volunteers (CSVs) to look after the needs of severely disabled people, living with them at home or visiting frequently. There are also examples of disabled people receiving direct grants from local authorities which they can use to employ their own carers or other help. This gives them the maximum of control over their own care arrangements.

Individual members of MACC explain the reasons which led them to join the group. The Neighbourhood Care Groups' co-ordinator at the CVS thinks that 'institutional care can't be right on a long-term basis – it's so dehumanising'. The CVS development officer feels strongly that 'people should be able to live lives of equal status and equal value as able-bodied/-minded people in the community'. She sees personal dignity as very important, and points to the need for flexible services with a completely different attitude from the uncaring or patronising one so often displayed towards elderly and disabled people.

With these issues in mind, the alliance produced a Manifesto setting out its aims, and called a launch meeting in 1982. Since then, the group has met regularly, usually on a monthly basis (with sub-groups also operating), and has consisted of around ten people.

Funding and resources

MACC has never had any resources of its own: the CVS and CHC have financed mailings and publications. Members have incorporated some work for MACC into their own jobs, and have given some time voluntarily. However, the volume of work has increased considerably and the group is arranging to apply for funding for a full-time worker.

Objective

The Manifesto describes MACC's objective as 'to support positively the right of people in Manchester who are disabled by age, or by physical or mental impairment, to live and participate in the community'. Rather than seeing residential hostels as the only alternative to hospitals, MACC exists to press for the development of community facilities with a radically different approach. The need for individual choice is emphasised, with 'a variety of different housing types', 'a range of non-residential support services including carers, medical and nursing staff and domestic staff', and 'access to ... employment, recreational, educational and transport services'. Relatives, too, should have a choice about how much to take part in caring.

MACC wishes to perform a liaison and information function: consulting voluntary organisations, consumers, relatives, professionals and staff groups about their views, through mailings and open meetings, and keeping them in touch with national and local developments in the community care programme. MACC also campaigns amongst health authorities and local authorities for its objectives to be implemented.

Activities

Accountability to consumers

MACC is very concerned that services should be planned in consultation with the consumers who will use them. For example, people who are going to live in a house should be involved in its design. At present, this happens only rarely. Two local consumers were invited to speak at the launch meeting of MACC: Frank Tranter, who is severely disabled and lives at home with the help of his wife, community nurses and community service volunteers, and Kenny Spurrell, who used to live in a hostel and now lives with others in his own home. Their talks, which described what it felt like to be on the receiving end of the services, were then published by MACC in a pamphlet entitled *Inside Out*. MACC is presently trying to decide whether consumers should become members of the MACC group itself, or whether it is better to arrange some other form of liaison.

Open meetings

MACC holds open meetings on particular topics, which have been fairly well attended, and have given smaller groups a useful chance to exchange views and to find out how planning systems work.

Keeping in touch with local projects

MACC does not itself run projects; it is a pressure and liaison group. However, the ideas discussed at MACC meetings are often based on members' experience in or knowledge of particular community care projects. Several local projects provide useful models for the way in which community care could evolve. (The projects mentioned here are just a few examples of the many and varied areas in which MACC members are working.)

For example, Outreach is a community-based organisation which provides services for people with special needs, including people with mental handicaps. Its activities include running a weekly social club, and volunteers regularly accompany small groups of people to the pub, disco or cinema, so that they can learn how to use the facilities, and practise the skills of relating to others.

The alliance has become interested in 'advocacy', in which volunteers befriend disabled people and speak out on their behalf where appropriate: for example, to make sure that they get the welfare benefits they are entitled to. After sounding out the opinions of local organisations, the alliance applied for a grant from Manchester Health Authority for a worker to set up an advocacy scheme in Higher Blackley, to help mentally handicapped people to use leisure facilities. This scheme is operating independently of MACC.

There are 23 Neighbourhood Care Groups in the Manchester area. The co-ordinator of the groups explains that all share the aim of helping people to live in the community. The groups relieve the burden on carers by finding people to take over for a while. Some groups have a drop-in session, and others arrange home visits. Paid workers should provide the main input, but family, friends, neighbours and volunteers could all be involved. Most Care Groups think that their time is best used for befriending, rather than for tasks such as bathing people and cleaning, which they see as the responsibility of the statutory services.

104

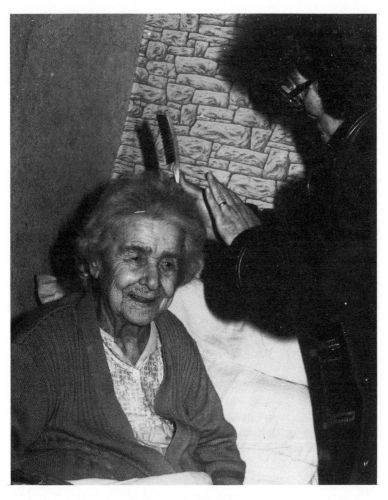
Community care in Manchester

The Association of Carers, an organisation particularly aware of the position of women as carers, has set up a local branch in Manchester. As well as giving help to individual carers, the association brings them together to press for changes in government policy which will improve their lives financially and practically. Such issues, raised in the Equal Opportunities Commission report on the status of carers, have been discussed within MACC.

Housing needs

The availability of suitable housing is a basic requirement for progressive forms of community care. Some housing associations in Manchester are already having discussions with interested voluntary groups, and/or with the hospitals whose patients will be coming into the community. As a contribution to the debate, and as a general educational tool, MACC has produced a tape-slide programme about the right of everyone to live in their own homes rather than in institutions.

Contact with the statutory services

The statutory services have traditionally seen the voluntary sector as a useful service provider, but voluntary groups have rarely been formally consulted by official planning committees. In Manchester, a recent series of meetings convened by the statutory authorities brought together representatives of social services, the three district health authorities and voluntary organisations, to discuss how 'Care in the Community' could be put into practice. The North West Regional Health Authority is lending money to districts, which is supposed to cover the costs of bringing mentally handicapped people out of hospital. The amount will be £10,800 per person per year. This money is not yet available for other groups such as elderly or mentally ill people. The city council and the health districts fear that the money is not going to be enough. Some people might require less than the £10,800 per year, but others could need much more. The city council's finances are precarious, since it recently lost £250 million in government grants.

Voluntary groups are being invited to put forward grant applications for back-up schemes for community care. The statutory services appreciate the support that voluntary groups can give, but are concerned that voluntary organisations might take on massive schemes for resettling people in the community, which later will have to be funded by the social services.

MACC has taken a leading role in bringing voluntary

organisations together to campaign effectively at this key moment. MACC has convened a series of meetings for voluntary organisations, so that opinions on community care can be discussed in preparation for joint meetings with the statutory sector. Many people present felt that the Government programme was too hurried and was designed to produce cuts, that there was already insufficient community care provision, that the burden would fall on relatives and friends as well as on social services, and that relatives must be consulted before people left hospital. It was also argued that money should be made available for all groups needing facilities, not only for the mentally handicapped.

The voluntary sector meetings have drawn up detailed proposals for the election of voluntary organisation representatives on to Joint Care Planning Teams and Joint Consultative Committees. They have emphasised the need for a proper structure for elections, and for finance to be provided in order to enable voting and administration to take place. At a workshop on 25 May 1983, those present gave the alliance a mandate to continue negotiations on behalf of voluntary organisations in Manchester, 61 of which are affiliated to MACC.

The voluntary sector is diverse and groups have many different views: it is hard to produce coherent policies. Structures are also needed to make sure that people speaking on behalf of voluntary organisations are accountable to the people they represent. MACC's funding application for a full-time worker envisages that the person appointed would spend considerable time on facilitating liaison between voluntary groups, and developing the process of representation.

Responses to official documents

MACC has responded to documents on community care, produced locally and nationally. The community health council automatically receives a large number of these; for example, MACC commented on a North West Regional Health Authority document on 'A Model District Service for Mentally Handicapped People'. Some officials may actually welcome comments on their circulars: one telephoned from London, keen to talk to the Manchester Disability Forum.

MACC has written to point out that Government circulars on Care in the Community are unrealistic, since the necessary finance is not forthcoming. Another national move has been to ask MPs to raise questions in the House of Commons about the resources being put into community care. Ministers are then required to consult the DHSS for replies.

Are the objectives being achieved?

Some, though by no means all, of the facilities currently operating in Manchester already do meet MACC's criteria for good standards of community care. However, it seems that ideas about community care are changing. The principle that disabled people *can* live normally in the community, for example in schemes such as Core and Cluster, is more widely accepted now. Many people attending MACC's workshops have found the discussion stimulating. Through MACC's information work, voluntary groups are now more aware that chronically ill and disabled people will soon be coming out into the community. The voluntary sector is also better equipped with ideas on what the different possibilities for community care might be, as shown in the tape-slide on independent living.

MACC has been instrumental in negotiating the format of voluntary organisation representation on the Joint Care Planning Teams which formulate the proposals discussed by JCCs.

Lessons learned

Developing new ideas on community care can be a slow process. The greatest resistance to the idea of disabled people coming into the community sometimes comes from parents and relatives. Parents of patients aged 20–30 made the decision to put their children in hospital many years ago, at a time when there were few community facilities available. Families believed that they were acting in their sons and

108

daughters' best interests, and suddenly to have their decision questioned can engender a lot of guilt. Many parents feel that their sons and daughters *need* to be dependent, or are not able to live independent lives.

Other parents may have doubts as to whether the community can provide good quality care for their sons and daughters. Calderstones, a mental handicap hospital close to Manchester, is due to close, and the parents' group is worried about their sons and daughters coming out of hospital to a family and a community without enough resources. Community care may mean a greater burden on relatives. As one member of MACC asks:

> How *do* you exonerate the family? They are bound to experience pressure. It's rather simple to say 'we'll bring your son or daughter into the community and you won't have to do anything'. Either they will end up doing it or they'll feel guilty for *not* doing it.

She then goes on to point out the possible pitfalls of 'independent living'. Some people who have developed relationships with hospital staff over many years may suddenly find themselves alone in the community. They may have well-equipped housing, but little contact with people: 'It's not enough to have a flat full of gadgets and know how to use them. You also need to know how to use social facilities and build up friendship networks.' Perhaps MACC should concentrate on ensuring that there is enough support for people already in the community, before more come out of hospital.

Another member thinks that MACC could end up adopting too inflexible an approach to housing in the community: 'We could set up a new model – "Everybody has to live in four-bedroomed houses", for example. It could be a new form of institution, repeating the feeling of no choice.' He is interested in the Neighbourhood Network Scheme in Bolton, in which mentally handicapped people are resettled with appropriate staff living nearby. The person's needs are assessed first, rather than allocating the most suitable housing regardless of its location and its social networks. In one case in the Bolton scheme, a nurse had two mentally handi-

109

capped young men living with him, an arrangement which seemed to suit all of them.

Health service unions have given a lukewarm response to the community care programme, since jobs are likely to be lost when institutions close. Even if workers are offered alternative jobs, such as being care assistants, they may be required to move to a different area.

On the issue of the reorganisation of existing schemes, things may be more hopeful. Hostels presently run as institutions could perhaps have smaller living groups, each with their own staff. It is often said that staff do not want any changes in the demarcation of their jobs. However, in a discussion with a regional officer from one union, MACC found that staff are rarely consulted. Some changes have in fact taken place with staff agreement. In the future, MACC hopes to contact unions for further discussion.

Could an organisation like MACC be set up elsewhere? The voluntary sector in Manchester is strong and well organised, with many funded workers who can give time and resources to an organisation such as MACC. These conditions may not apply elsewhere. The MACC group has included three local councillors: although they have not attended in that capacity, they have been well informed about local authority committees and planning systems. This is also unlikely to be typical.

An essential ingredient of MACC's success is a high degree of trust. Members of MACC have always been willing to listen to each other's ideas and discuss different topics: participants note that nobody's complained about being left out or said 'I'm not interested in that area.' Meetings have been informal, with decisions reached by consensus. People have attended MACC as interested individuals, not as representatives of particular organisations.

It is an achievement that a group of people in the voluntary sector has managed to work together productively without a formal structure. This has probably been possible because MACC's members share similar ideas on community care issues, a bond which might not have been discovered if Manchester CVS had not called that first meeting.

110